# A HISTORY
## *of the*
# ISLE OF WIGHT
# HOSPITALS

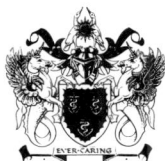

# A HISTORY
## *of the*
# ISLE OF WIGHT
# HOSPITALS

*by E. F. Laidlaw*

PUBLISHED BY CROSS PUBLISHING
NEWPORT, ISLE OF WIGHT

*Dedicated to all who have worked, who work now*
*or who will work in the future at*
*St. Mary's Hospital*

Front cover plate. A ward scene - probably about 1900.
*Courtesy: R. Brinton.*
Back cover plate. Main entrance to the House of Industry.
*Courtesy: J. & J. Jones and Dovecote Press.*

# CONTENTS

# LIST OF PLATES

# LIST OF FIGURES

# FOREWORD

Dr Eric Laidlaw provides a series of fascinating snapshots of an important aspect of the Island's history. A comprehensive description of the development of the varied hospital buildings is enlivened by vivid references to the day to day problems of patients, staff and administrators. Coping with epidemics, infection, injury and mental illness against a background of daunting social conditions but nobly assisted by the benevolence of local people of goodwill, is illuminated by the author's affection for his topic.

Echoing throughout this lucid review is the finding that hospitals become obsolete for the demands placed upon them between their planning and official opening. The endless struggle to cope with this problem continues to the present day. Throughout the history of the services, the explosion of medical and nursing skills, development of drugs, ancillary and pathological and radiological services together with the rising expectations of patients and an aging population will ensure that the dilemma continues.

The author has laid down a valuable database to which future managers of health services may refer with profit.

B. Livesey, C.B., F.R.C.S

# PREFACE

The suggestion that I should write this book was made to me in the winter of 1993 by Mr. Tony Blee, then the General Administrator of the Isle of Wight Health Authority; and later the St. Mary's Trust kindly agreed to sponsor me and to pay part of the expenses. I am duly grateful to both the Trust and Mr. Blee and most especially to Major-General Brian Livesey for writing a foreword.

The most important source of information has been from the minutes and reports of the Councils, Committees and Boards which managed the various hospitals, which up to about 1970 are mostly housed in the County Records Office and I am glad to thank the staff of that office who have carried so many heavy tomes from one room to another for me; also Audrey Elliot of Medina Borough Council, who helped me to hunt, with limited success, for the records of the Borough Councils of past years, and to Mavis Granger who has led me around the circumference of Whitecroft where records of the last 25 years are, with luck, to be found; and has found me vicarious accommodation where I might study them.

Another important source of information available at the Records Office has been past numbers of the *County Press* over the last century or so and of early Ordnance Survey maps; and in the County Library an earlier paper the *County Observer,* and various books, especially Worsley's History of the Island and the book *An Illustrated History of the Isle of Wight* by J. & J. Jones; also Cooke's *A New Picture of the Isle of Wight;* Bill Shepard's *Newport Remembered;* Mr. A. Parker's two short books about Shanklin, and Cantwell and Sprack on *The Solent Defences*, but apart from this official or printed information, I have in the course of two years received advice and help from so many different people that I could not give a complete list of them and I would like to take this opportunity to thank them all collectively here; there are some that I must mention individually, - Mrs. Margham; Miss Sylvia White; Miss Weedon and Miss Johnson, all of whom remember the coming of the N.H.S. at Newport, Mr. Rouse, the former Chief Engineer who typed out for me an account of the building and engineering work at St. Mary's while he was there; Jack Keech who was Secretary of St. Mary's for many years and Bruce Charman who was secretary at Whitecroft and later took Mr. Keech's place at St. Mary's; Mr. Hunt, the only man I have spoken to who worked at St. Mary's before it became a hospital and was in fact assistant to the Master of the House of Industry and who later became assistant to Jack Keech; Mrs. Elizabeth (Heather) Gray and others from the Frank James staff and Mrs. Eileen Down; Mrs. Phillips, who had nursing experience in both world wars in the emergency hospitals, Dr David Cooper, who gave me details of Parkhurst Prison Hospital and Dr P.D. Swinstead, retired consultant Pathologist. Apart from those associated with the hospital, I must thank Mr. Roy Brinton and Mr. A. Gale who have given me much information about Ryde in particular, and Mr. E.H. Burbridge who gave me an account of St. Catherine's Home in Ventnor.

The history of the hospitals seems to divide itself naturally into two parts. Up to 1948 each hospital had its own management board or committee and after 1948 when there was one central organisation, and I have divided the book accordingly.

Where I have referred to money matters, - income, expenditure, prices, charges, costs, etc. I have used the units in use at the time, that is for the most part the old L.S.D. style. It is usually of course only the pounds that matter and I have generally when extracting figures from records given them to the nearest pound; but occasionally shillings and pence seem worth recording.

In the course of preparing this book I have of course encountered a great many names of administrators, doctors, matrons, nurses, hospital servants, members of committees, Medical Officers, Councillors and especially givers of various bounties. Many names come up naturally in the course of the story, but I regret many that I have not mentioned, including many who were well known in their day and many still well known now. There may be some who feel surprise or even disappointment that their own name, or some other particular names, are not mentioned. To these I can only apologise for my omission.

Such maps and plans as I have been able to produce come mostly from Ordnance Survey Maps; there have been a very few plans available of buildings at St. Mary's, and one very early one of Ryde Hospital, for which my thanks are due to Mr. R. Brinton.

It is a pleasure to acknowledge with thanks the reliable and painstaking work of Tina Snow in producing the type-script and the ever ready help and advice in word and deed of Mr. Peter Cross and his staff, Anita Govinden and Marion Giddings.

Finally with all my heart I thank my step-son, Robin McInnes for help and advice especially about the illustrations and my wife Brenda for her endurance, tolerance and help, and her good memory.

# PART ONE

*From the beginning to 1948*

# I

## INTRODUCTION

In the census of 1851, a year or so after the opening of the Ryde Hospital (known then as the Royal Isle of Wight Infirmary), the population of the Island was 45,640; it had increased, indeed nearly doubled, since the first census in 1801 when it was 23,687; and the figure for 1771, the year of the foundation of the House of Industry which became St. Mary's, estimated from the returns of the parishes, was 18,700.

As to doctors the earliest figures I have been able to get were from the local list in the Medical Directory of 1848; at this time there were 33 doctors on the Island; if we consider only General Practitioners, the proportion of doctors to population is not so very different from the present.

Medicine and surgery were about to develop rapidly; anaesthesia had been introduced during the previous few years and the possibilities of surgery were thereby very greatly extended; up until then, surgery must have been mostly concerned with injuries, broken limbs, war wounds; hernias and other local swellings and superficial growths and infections; and cutting for stone. Medicine must have dealt mainly with infectious diseases especially Cholera, Smallpox, Typhoid Fever, and Typhus, Scarlet Fever, Pneumonia, Erysipelas, and others including Tuberculosis. Other diseases and disorders, - Parkinsonism, - the Shaking Palsy, Multiple Sclerosis, - the Creeping Palsy, Strokes, Apoplexy, Gout, Rheumatism and Arthritis, Epilepsy, Diabetes were known, but there was no systematic knowledge of medicine based upon human anatomy and physiology; the first treatise of Human Histology (The Microscopic Structure of Tissues and Organs) was published by Arthur Hill Hassall in 1849, and the first edition of *Gray's Anatomy* was in 1858. The work of Pasteur & Lister and the recognition of micro-organisms as a cause of disease, was still about two decades in the future.

There was however a medical service of some sort; the Board of Guardians which was responsible for the House of Industry, also provided a medical and nursing service for those who could not pay. From 1836 onwards the Guardians were responsible to the Poor Law Board, which sent inspectors annually to report on the Workhouse. But the Guardians operated before 1836, - the leading landowners and clerics of the Island, - 'The Oligarchy of Gentlemen' as J. & J. Jones have described them, - and it was in 1830 that Mr. Sewell suggested that the Island be divided into ten areas; to each one a doctor was to be appointed; they varied in size and population and were to be chosen by the doctors in their order of seniority in the profession; their salaries were to be proportional to the population in their area, and ranged from £25 p.a. to £95 p.a.; and as will be seen later a doctor was also appointed to the House of Industry and one to the associated wards for the mentally afflicted; we may assume that all these were part-time appointments, these arrangements were made for those who could not pay. The scheme unfortunately did not work very well, perhaps partly because of the extremely isolated condition and situation of the South Wight, most especially of the Undercliff. At the end of a year or two, five areas were vacant. Many re-arrangements were made, but the principle remained that some sort of salaried service was provided for the poor.

The Guardian's medical services also included the provision of dispensaries. The first of these, in Castlehold, Newport, was opened in 1823; a surgeon (doctor) attended between 8 a.m. and 10 a.m.; by 1832, about the same time as the ten areas were designated, the Guardians ordained three dispensaries in each of the east and west Medines; accommodation was to be provided, and one supposes maintained, by the Guardians, and medicines by the doctors; each dispensary was to be visited daily; parish overseers were authorised to send a pauper with messages, and to bring back medicines prescribed. A dispensary in Ryde was started in 1842 and was ultimately housed at the junction of West Street and Swanmore Road close to the Hospital which in 1952 finally took it over. The headquarters of the Ryde Red Cross now occupies the site of the former dispensary.

Some years before that in 1826 it was thought that the midwives on the Island were too few in number, and surgeons were asked to find four eligible women who were to go to London for training and return to the Island to practice; they would receive 5 shillings for each case they delivered successfully.

The practice of medicine at the higher levels in those days demanded an astonishingly comprehensive understanding of philosophy and logic; Dr Gray in his biographical study of Arthur Hill Hassall *By Candle-light*, describes the examination for the London M.D. in 1847, which includes a written paper on *Elements of intellectual philosophy, logic and moral philosophy*; how, one wonders would today's membership candidates deal with such questions as 'There are, and can be, but two ways of investigating truth. What are these two methods and what is the difference between them as regards the process of the mind?' or 'Give Stewart's definition of consciousness. How according to him do we get the notion and conviction of our personal identity? Give any other solution of the question.' or 'What are the presumptions that we shall live after death deduced from our present physical, intellectual and moral state?' (These are three of the twelve questions posed.)

What happened to patients in need of hospital care before there was a General Hospital on the Island? The only hospital available in those early years was the County Hospital in Winchester; patients could be taken there, but the number able to make the journey and to benefit must have been very small, and the difficulties formidable; the regular service from Cowes to Southampton only began in the mid 19th century; and the journey from Southampton to Winchester must have had to be on horse-back or by a horse-drawn carriage of some sort until the railways came into existence also in the mid century. Nevertheless, a few did find their way there and Guardians were authorised to arrange this and to accompany a patient to Winchester, and to be reimbursed the expense of the journey and return.

It is perhaps a little unexpected to find that the hospitals which eventually came into being on the Island numbered so many as (about) 20, though it is true that some of them need only a very brief mention. Besides the general hospitals we have to consider the special hospitals, Whitecroft, the R.N.H., Longford, and Ashey; three small fever or isolation hospitals besides the larger one at Fairlee; Frank James and the three small Shanklin hospitals, - the Cottage Hospital, the Arthur Webster Institute and Scio House; the military and naval hospitals; and the prison hospital and some others that had only a very brief existence. During the two world wars several of the big houses were taken over as service hospitals or convalescent homes, these included Ryde House, Ryde Castle, Gatcombe, Swainston, Afton Manor, Northwood House and Winchester House in Lake and Haslewood in Ryde and there were of course, and are, numerous convalescent homes and nursing homes some of which have been more or less closely associated with the hospital work - Ryde Nursing Home, for example and Kitehill Nursing Home. The Harriet Guy and Cowes War Memorial Convalescent Home was given as an endowment for public service; whilst Osborne House has been a convalescent home since the beginning of the century available for a limited range of the public, but giving great help to the hospital service during the wars.

St. Catherine's Home in Ventnor also requires special mention; it opened as a nursing home for adults in 1879, founded by a committee with the support of the C of E Convent of St. Margaret at East Grinstead, this association continued, and until the modern era it cared mainly for adults and children with respiratory illnesses.

In 1910 it became a childrens' home, increasing in size by building and taking in adjacent houses, and ultimately having as many as 150 children of which 120 were boys, 30 girls. During the Second World War about a third of the children moved to the Hermitage, at the back of St. Catherine's Hill.

Hospitals necessarily work in co-operation with other medical services, - general practice and public health - and any account of hospitals cannot be separated entirely from these; up to 1948 most of the senior staff in the hospitals were also in general or specialist practice independent of their hospital duties; and the County Medical Officer and his staff controlled St. Mary's Hospital and Longford until 1948; several clinics were housed in County Hall even after 1948 for a few years, and there was constant communication between the County Medical Officer and hospital workers and authorities; and the county provided a district nursing service and of course the nursing staff for its own hospitals, and was concerned with nurse training in the hospitals. Consequently, although I do not attempt to give a history of medical and nursing services on the Island, it is impossible not to mention them from time to time.

The very first hospital on the Island, not yet mentioned, must of course have been the Leper Hospital at Gunville in the 13th century, associated with St. Augustine's Priory at Carisbrooke from which monks visited the nearby hospital regularly. Father Hockey wrote that a monk from St. Augustine's celebrated mass there three times a week; and that Isabella de Fortibus when she was the owner of the Island made it a regular allowance of one silver mark yearly. Leper hospitals in those days probably accepted a number of other disorders associated with skin rashes; Leprosy itself was quite uncommon. Father Hockey moreover mentions that the accounts of the hospital reveal that over a period of a year in 1312 only one single patient, on an average, was resident in the hospital. I do not know when this hospital closed down; if it survived until the dissolution of the monasteries, it would have had a longer life than any other hospital on the Island has had as yet.

The history of hospitals on the Island obviously can only enter occasionally and tangentially into the wider history of the towns in which they were built or of the Island itself. I hope I have been able to say enough, here and there, to indicate some of the developing scene and the ideas, the problems and activities of the people, - our forebears of five and six generations - who, although their life-styles over the years may have been very different from ours, were not themselves less intelligent, thoughtful, considerate, or at times bewildered than their descendants. The new hospitals are built figuratively or sometimes literally on the foundations of the old and we stand on the shoulders of those who created them.

# II

# ROYAL ISLE OF WIGHT COUNTY HOSPITAL
## 1849 TO 1992

On Tuesday, September 28th 1848, a general meeting of subscribers to the Royal I.o.W. Infirmary was held in Newport Town Hall; the Mayor of Newport, James Eldridge, was in the Chair, and he called upon Col. Harcourt, later M.P. for the Island in 1851-52, to read the draft of the proposed statutes of the Infirmary. These specified that the Management was to be in the hands of the Governors 'As qualified hereinafter'. The hospital was to be for the relief of the sick and disabled poor from all parts of the Island. Admission however would be dependent upon the patient procuring a letter of recommendation from a subscriber, except in the case of sudden accident or emergency - all such urgent cases would be received at any hour of the day or night.

The Management Committee was to be composed of twelve governors, with a Chairman; three were to retire each year, - but could be re-appointed. There were to be weekly meetings of the Committee and accounts were to be rendered monthly. The Committee would have the authority to discharge Matron or House Surgeon for misconduct and to appoint temporary officers in their place; that apart, control of the hospital was to be exclusively in the hands of the Governors, but the committee would submit their recommendations. The Queen had already consented to be the Patron, - hence the justification for the Royal title; the President was Lord Yarborough.

The subscribers of 2 guineas became Governors for a year; and those of 20 guineas became life Governors. (We must remember that 2 guineas in those days was in terms of purchasing power the equivalent of at least £100 now and 20 guineas, £1000.)

This was not, obviously, the first meeting intending to plan the hospital; much had already been done and there had been a committee which had met probably on at least half a dozen occasions and which had produced the draft. But it does seem to have been the first meeting which is recorded in the archives of the hospital. There had been meetings certainly in 1845 and 1847 when much of the preliminary planning had been settled. By April 1847, Thomas Hellyer of Ryde had been appointed Honorary Architect and was made a life Governor. He had submitted a design for a 20 bedded hospital which had been accepted and was estimated to cost £1,630-11s-6d. Messrs Jolliffe had been appointed builders, and J. Percival Esq. of Woodlands, Treasurer. It was estimated that the cost of running the hospital would be £300 per 10 beds per annum.

Among the pioneers of these earlier meetings were Rev. W. Spencer Phillips, Rector of Newchurch, and a surgeon, Mr. A.T.S. Dodd. Newchurch in those days was a parish which stretched from shore to shore and included Ryde and Ventnor; but the Rector had realised that a large part of his flock lived in Ryde, and Ryde was chosen as the most suitable site for a hospital since it was said to be within 12 miles of four fifths of the Islands population (which must still be the case) and was also suitable for hot and cold sea baths. At the meeting in 1845, £400 had already been subscribed and by 1847 £1250; land for the hospital had been made available by Miss Player and Miss Brigstocke who provided it at a nominal rent for 99 years; later, about the turn of the century, extended to 999 years.

Among the conditions laid down in the draft now read, it was required that the House Surgeon and Matron, and nurses and servants, all of whom would be resident 'Shall be unmarried, or in such circumstances as not to be inconvenienced with the care of a family'. And that patients 'Such as are discharged, cured or relieved, shall be enjoined by the Committee to return thanks in their respective places of worship, and also to the persons who recommended them to the Infirmary; for both of which purposes printed papers shall be delivered to them'. There were to be strictly no gratuities - on pain of immediate discharge if a patient, or dismissal if on the staff. More suggestive of modern times perhaps were the conditions that all complaints were to be notified to the Committee; and visitors wishing to inspect the Infirmary might do so at appointed times.

There might need to be a waiting list for admissions. The House Surgeon might reject unsuitable patients, informing the subscriber by letter; after a patient had been in the hospital for three months the Committee might discharge him or her unless the Medical Officer desired otherwise; in which case a further letter of recommendation must be obtained. In the case of death, the subscriber or the patient's friends, or parish, were expected to pay the funeral expenses, which in no case should be more than 30s; the expenses of transport home must in the case of patients coming from a distance be provided by the subscriber. Any soldier admitted must have payment guaranteed by his officer. Patients discharged for irregularity should never be re-admitted unless by special consent of the Committee.

The first meeting of the Governors was held in October 1849 just a year or so after this inaugural meeting; with James Player Lind in the chair; the Vice-Presidents included Captain T.R. Brigstocke, John Hamborough and Sir William Oglander Bt. The Honorary Chaplain was the Rev. Laurence Tuttiett; Dr Martin of Ventnor was appointed Honorary Consultant Physician and Mr. Richard Bloxam, Consultant Surgeon; there were to be four Medical Officers, B. Barrow, R.W. Bloxam, Henry Phene and T. Bell-Salter. The Medical Officer on duty was an ex-officio member of the Committee. The House Surgeon who was also to serve as Secretary was appointed and the first Matron was a Miss Pascoe.

Several categories of patients were excluded, - not to be admitted; namely those with Consumption; Smallpox; Venereal Disease; Epilepsy; and the Itch; and also those considered incurable; the insane; those with inoperable cancer; women with advanced pregnancy; and children under seven.

The minutes of this meeting included a final sentence 'Of the several reports, six in all, which have been published and circulated with the respect to the progress of the Royal Isle of Wight Infirmary, the last, issued by the late Committee on January 1849 was the first which contained a Debtor and Creditor account and was therefore, - as such statements of accounts will afterwards appear annually, - styled the first "Annual Report".'

There was reference at this meeting to a grand bazaar held in aid of the Infirmary by invitation of Col. and Lady Catherine Harcourt at St. Claire (now the St. Claire Holiday Camp); this had been attended by the Queen and members of the Royal Family; it had produced £847 which was said to be far in excess of the most sanguine expectation; (£800 in 1913 would according to Whitakers Almanac have had approximately the purchasing power of £40,000 now; - how much more £800 might have been in 1849 I do not know, - but it was indeed an impressive sum).

The report included a long list of rules for the Medical Officers, the House Surgeon and for the Secretary, Treasurer, Chaplain, Matron, nurses and servants. The M.Os. were to attend in a rota, one at 9 o'clock and one at ten o'clock on Mondays, Tuesdays, Thursdays and Saturdays. No Medical Officer was to prescribe for or intermeddle (sic) with the patients of any other M.O. except by his desire. No one should be allowed to see the prescription, practice or operations of the Medical Officers without their consent. No 'capital operation' was to be performed except in urgent cases without a consultation of Medical Officers and a Medical Officer was to attend each weekly Committee meeting to receive and examine patients recommended and certify his opinion of the cases and take them under his care if admitted.

The House Surgeon was to have under his care all medical stores, surgical instruments and pharmaceutical apparatus; keep an inventory and see that they were kept in good condition; on no account to lend any without written order from an Honorary Medical Officer, and when lent, take care that they were returned as soon as possible and fit for use. He was not allowed to entertain any party either for pleasure or for any other purpose within the house. The Matron was to have the keys of the outer doors and to lock up every evening at nine in the winter and ten in the summer.

For the servants the first requirement was that 'They should behave with kindness to the patients and with civility and respect to the officers of the establishment'. Finally the patients were to 'Wash their hands and faces every morning; to be decent and regular in their conduct; and not to swear nor use any improper language'. It is easy for us to smile at these rules; perhaps however we should recognise that they reflected the principles and practices of the time, - and who shall say that those of our own time are any better.

The hospital opened on November 9th 1849, - this date was chosen being the birthday of the Prince of Wales. There were now 25 beds rather than 20, 5 being set aside for paying patients or other purposes; in the first year, - that is up to the presentation of the second Annual Report to the A.G.M. in 1850, there had been 83 in-patients and 37 out-patients; the number, especially of out-patients rose rapidly; 125 in-patients and 457 out-patients in 1850-51, and - to anticipate - after 25 years, in 1874-75 there were 293 in-patients and 1547 out-patients. Much happened during those 25 years and indeed afterwards; the minutes indicate the main concerns of the Committee, the Governors and Medical Officers, dealing chiefly with admissions and discharges, subscriptions and donations, governorships; collections in churches and elsewhere, appointments and changes of staff; day to day maintenance; catering and house keeping; and new buildings; and there was a variety of incidental matters, some of which may be of some interest and throw light upon the times. In 1850, a special meeting of Governors considered the admission of patients from the Middlesex Hospital for the purpose of sea bathing; this was to be allowed on payment of such sum as would fully cover all expenses and provided that 20 beds remained for Isle of Wight patients; in 1851 the occupation of Turnpike Cottage was considered, this was a cottage situated adjacent to the main entrance, as it then was, to the hospital, which became the exit for cars and other wheeled traffic. The cottage, I think, must have been demolished because a lodge was later built close to that site. In 1852 the creation of a Public House almost opposite the Infirmary was to be opposed by every means in the power of the Committee (in parenthesis it seems fair to say that one is not aware of any adverse influence exerted by 'The London' on the hospital; possibly at times the juxta-position was, to some on both sides, convenient. The old 'London' of course is gone now replaced by the new one.

In 1855 six beds were set aside for soldiers invalided from the Crimean War; this was later increased to 12 (the Government to pay) and in that year the Chairman of the Governors wrote to the Master of the Workhouse in Newport asking if he could recommend a nurse for the female ward; in 1856 there was a problem about the admission of the wives and children of soldiers at Albany Barracks in Parkhurst, a problem which recurred several times over the years.

There were staff problems; the H.S. in post at the time of the opening was apparently not acceptable to the M.Os. and Governors; he left and a Mr. Billinghurst, or one of the Honorary M.Os., undertook to fulfil all H.S. duties for a month until someone else could be appointed; advertisements were placed in the *Lancet* and the *Medical Times*. In 1856 a disagreement between the Matron and the House Surgeon led to the latter resigning; in the following year Col. Harcourt reported to the Committee that he had encountered the Matron unfit for duty having over indulged herself; she resigned the next week. (This was not Miss Pascoe who had moved on earlier). In 1854 the advertisement for a House Surgeon offered the post to 'A legally qualified gentleman', - He would be required to act also as Secretary and to visit out-patients; (Home visiting seems to have been part of the House Surgeon's duties for several years to come, - even though he was the sole resident). In 1858 permission was given to George Dash, a porter (of whom more will be written later) to marry, provided that he lived at the lodge which was built for him; 10s-6d was allowed for his board wages. In 1859 the offer of a pew to be reserved in the parish church for the Medical Officer was declined; the Committee felt that in future a difference of creed of the M.O. might make the arrangement objectionable. In 1860 the porter, George Dash was given a key and a bell was fixed to ring in his lodge at night so that he could admit emergencies during the night.

In 1868 there was debate about the admission of the wives and families of policemen on the Island, - it was felt that with a salary of £1 weekly and free accommodation and medical care that they would not qualify as poor people needing free hospital care; they could no doubt have been admitted but would have to go into the paying patients beds.

In trying to give an account of the hospital's history it seems best to deal with it under several headings although of course it developed as a whole and the different headings are closely inter-related; viz Buildings, Management, Staff and Finance.

The earliest picture of the hospital about the time of its foundation shows the front recognisable with a main entrance looking East flanked by three tall windows on either side; a three storey building with the upper floor then having the appearance of attics with small windows; a ground plan about 1860 confirms this structure showing the main entrance connected with a cross corridor running from north to south with a set of rooms in the front and at the back. In 1851, however, Thomas Hellyer had added an Out-patients Department and a laundry and these also are shown on that plan; and about 1862 a lodge was built close to what is now the regular exit which must have involved the demolition of Turnpike Cottage. In 1864 Mr. Barrow, one of the Honorary Surgeons, reported that the wards were overcrowded, each bed having only 720 cubic feet of space, whereas 1,000 cubic feet was considered desirable; he suggested that some beds should be moved upstairs. However, at the time, the Committee was already advising the Governors to enlarge the buildings, and had approved plans for this. Again the plans were due to Thomas Hellyer who remained the Honorary Architect for about four decades; these additional buildings increased the maximum number of beds to 38. In 1857 gas lighting for the hospital was considered and shortly afterwards was installed at a cost of £16.

In 1870 the Medical Officers urged better accommodation for fevers and stressed the need for the nurses and a laundry relating to such cases to be kept separate; under pressure from them, the Chairman, Major Augustus Leeds, informed the Committee that he had entered into an agreement with a Mr. Austin for the purchase of a separate house for the reception of fever patients. The Chairman's action however was disputed, carried only by a small majority, but at the next meeting, a week later, rescinded and it was agreed that new wards should be built. At this time there was a Ryde Borough Council and it had created a sub-committee dealing with highways, gas and health and sanitary matters. This committee was interested in the provision of isolation wards for fevers and apparently would have undertaken part of the cost of patients admitted to such wards.

In January 1871 land was purchased for the new wards. The original plan seems to show the hospital grounds extending, as they now do, to the road immediately to the north of the hospital, Milligan Road then called Cemetery Road; but it seems that land for these wards which were to be built there had to be purchased by the Governors. It was suggested that these new wards should be a memorial to Sir John Simeon, and the Rev. Chisholm offered a

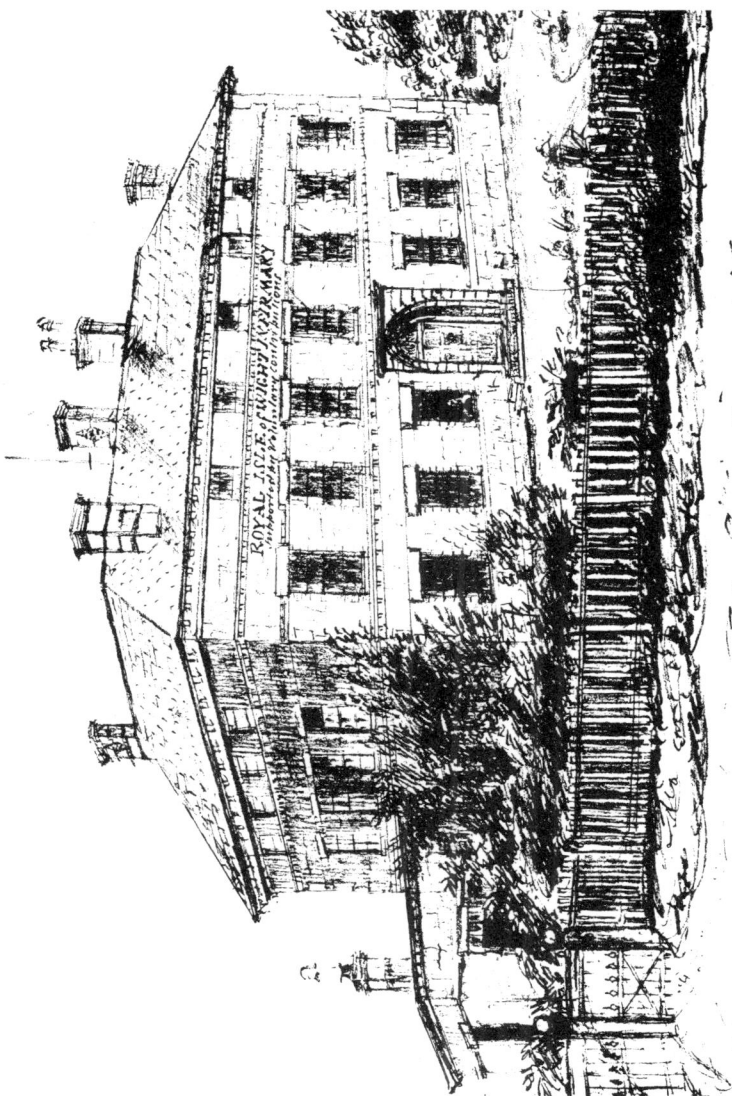

**Plate 1.** The Royal County Infirmary, about 1860. The upper floor at this stage must have provided rooms for nursing and domestic staff. The roof was raised about 1880. There was accommodation for 25 patients. The small building at the side was probably the Out-patient department: this and the laundry (at the back) were built in 1852. [See also figures 1, 2 & 3 pp 55, 56 & 57] *Courtesy: Dr Howell.*

subscription of up to £500 if this were agreed; however his family were unwilling to accept this form of memorial so that particular plan was abandoned; but the building of the wards was to go ahead.

In May of that year, 1871 the Sanitary Committee sought permission to build a temporary hospital in the grounds; but this was refused - it seems that it was to have been used for Smallpox.

The M.Os. were dissatisfied with the new wards when they were built. Mr. Barrow in particular who had persistently pressed for attention to drainage, ventilation and in general for a higher standard of accommodation, submitted his resignation in his displeasure but subsequently agreed to carry on; but he said that the wards were not as planned and the doctors with the support of J.B. Leeson Esq., M.D., F.R.C.P., F.R.S., of London complained that the design and ventilation of the wards was not satisfactory. The Architect submitted plans for enlargement and improvement of the wards and he also assured the Committee that the sanitation of the block was of the same pattern as that used in a series of well known buildings, mentioning the Radcliffe Infirmary at Oxford and the Institution of Mr. Eno the fruit salt manufacturer.

Meanwhile in 1874, Miss Lowther offered to raise £4,000 for a Childrens' Ward and Mr. Hellyer worked on a plan for this which the Committee asked the Governors to accept, and in 1877, Miss Milligan of East Ridge, Ryde proposed the erection of a convalescent home which was to be a memorial to her father and mother, - her father had fought in the Battle of Waterloo. This home was built and opened in 1881; Miss Milligan contributed in all about £5,500 towards its cost and endowment and its name is also associated with that of Marcus Lowther. It was known for a long time as the Milligan Convalescent Home or later as the Milligan Block and the institution was thereafter referred to as the Royal Isle of Wight Infirmary and Convalescent Home. It is of course the block lying to the West of the main hospital and opening onto West Street and it was connected to the main or central block of the hospital by a covered way and a flight of steps leading up to it; a memorial tablet is incorporated in the building and can still be seen above the entrance from West Street 'In Loving Memory of Robert and Elizabeth Milligan, this building is erected by their daughter Sophia Milligan 1880'.

The water supply to the hospital was derived at first from a well built close to what is now the main gateway which soon after the opening of the hospital had to be deepened but later the hospital went on to the main water supply. In those early times however George Dash had to pump water up into the storage tanks which would be presumably situated in the roof and which in the early days were of lead. These now, in 1881, were replaced by a galvanised iron tank and some years later the lead pipe supplying the tank was also replaced by a steel one.

Meanwhile in 1882 the roof of the original second floor was raised making the accommodation suitable for patients' wards; Mr. Barrow, now a member of the Committee and recently Mayor of Ryde after his retirement from the staff, asked for a communication between the fever wards and the main hospital; Mr. Hellyer indicated that he was planning a covered way and other modifications. A larger operating room was needed and a year or so later a new wing containing a sitting-room and three bedrooms for nurses as well as this operating room was built and also a new kitchen range and larder and a new ward with six beds for women together with a nurses' room and an enlarged dispensary and four additional bathrooms; by 1892 there were 50 beds plus 10 for fevers and 10 in the Convalescent Home; fire precautions were introduced with a hand engine which could be pulled along corridors and canvas shutes from the windows of the wards. (One hopes that patients never had to descend by these shutes). The need for more accommodation was persistent and about this time there was a project for a nurses' institution to be built in proximity to the hospital and Charles Seely M.P. offered £500 for this; but this plan did not come to fruition; it seems that the terms of the lease of the land did not allow such building on the hospital site and adjacent land was not found suitable. In 1894 plans for more accommodation for nurses and servants and for a lift were submitted; for the first time, the Architect now was not Thomas Hellyer who died that year; but by the next year, these things had been provided together with a new Consulting Room and a cabin for the porter within the building; and a new hot water system. Telephones were installed in 1898.

The most important and best known of the new buildings was to come in 1896 and the following years. Princess Henry of Battenberg, better known on the Island as Princess Beatrice, became Governor of the Island and President of the hospital in succession to her late husband who had died in Africa, in 1895; she supported the project to build a Childrens' Ward and expressed 'The earnest desire that it may be carried out as a memorial of Her Majesty's reign of 60 years'. The next year, 1897, she laid the foundation stone, albeit there was some concern about the diminution of (financial) support, and an interest free loan of £300 from E. Sweetman Esq., a member of the Committee was accepted.

The ward was designed by Messrs Young & Hall of Southampton Street, Bloomsbury, and built by Charles Langdon of Ryde. The opening by the Queen herself was on Friday July 19th 1899.

At 5.30 p.m. on that day, - half an hour before the time of the opening

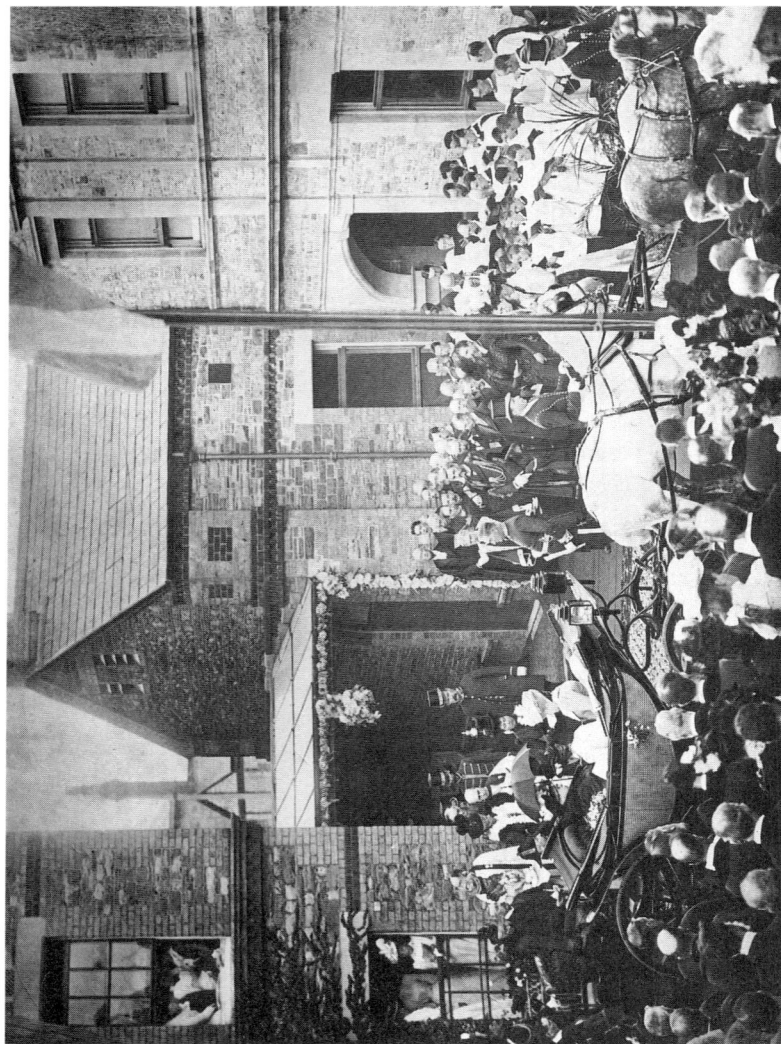

**Plate 2.** The Ceremonial Opening of Queen Victoria Ward. The Queen remained seated in her carriage (under a sun-shade): she was handed a disc with a switch which actuated the opening mechanism. The covered way, in time, became the entrance to the Casualty (A & E) department. *Courtesy: Roy Brinton.*

ceremony, - Princess Beatrice unveiled a bust of Queen Victoria, mounted above the ward and sculpted by E. Onslow-Forbes, R.A.; under it was the inscription 'Built and endowed as the Isle of Wight's commemoration of Queen Victoria's Diamond Jubilee. "She wrought her people lasting good" '.

The Queen's procession came into Ryde by Queen's Road and proceeded by John Street, the High Street, and Swanmore Road, and entered the hospital grounds by the new gate, where a Guard of Honour was drawn up; nurses and patients were assembled on the verandah in front of the hospital with the Matron, Miss Pinchard; and below the new ward were the boys from the Isle of Wight College. The Queen arrived at two minutes past 6.00 p.m. A short service was conducted by the Bishop, and the Queen, remaining in her coach, was then handed a silver disk which she pressed, thereby opening the doors of the ward.

The following day, Princess Beatrice accepted the ward on behalf of the Governors from the Commemoration Committee.

The Queen paid one more visit to the hospital in February 1900; it is said to have been one of the latest of her public engagements and was less than a year before her death. This seems to have been a quiet and unpublicised visit, and I cannot find any mention of it in the *County Press*; it was reported in *The Times* that the Queen had visited Queen Victoria Ward for Children at the RIoWCH; she was accompanied by Princess Henry of Battenberg and Princess Victoria of Schleswig-Holstein, and others, and was met and conducted to the ward by Dr A. Davey, the Rev. W. Welby, and Miss Skid, the Matron; there she distributed toys to the children. She returned from Osborne to Windsor shortly after this visit.

In 1903 a report was asked for from an independent Architect, T.W. Cutler, F.R.I.B.A. and when received must have caused some concern to the Committee, being rather highly critical. He said that the wards were divided into small rooms with the ventilation shared and heating inadequate; the theatre, kitchens, water closets and washrooms were in general bad; nurses' rooms lacked storage space; there was no cellar for wine and beer; no servants' hall; no porter's sitting-room; no Secretary's office; no visitors' waiting room; and no adequate system of ventilation and heating; no fire escape; and drainage was of doubtful efficiency. About the same time a Professor Colefield gave a report in which he considered that improved sanitation was absolutely necessary.

The Committee accepted Cutler's comments and a building sub-committee was formed and after discussions recommended Cutler's plans to the Committee. These involved the building of a 'sanitary tower', with some re-arrangement of the ground floor and the drainage; the provision of a fire escape; and the

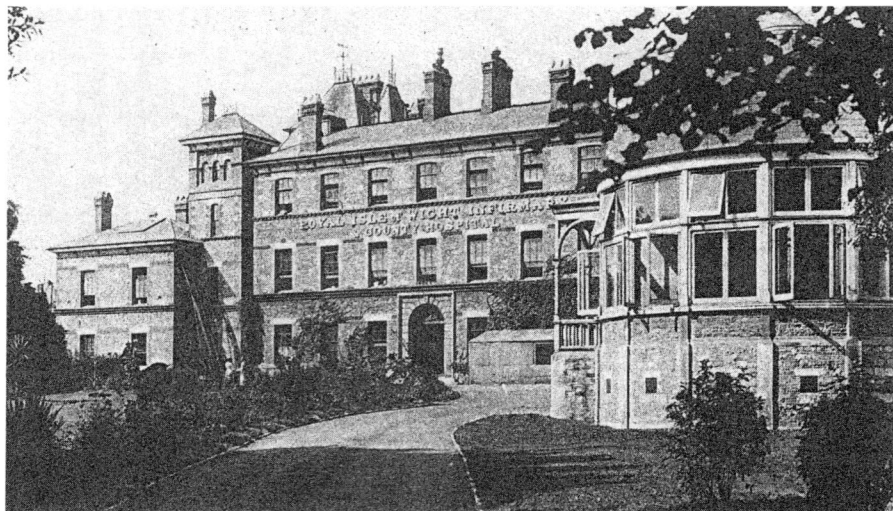

**Plate 3.** Royal Isle of Wight Infirmary. This must have been taken between 1899, when Victoria Ward on the right, was opened, and 1906 when the word Infirmary was removed from the hospital's title. There has been building on the far side, adding on to the original centre block, but the wards on that side have not yet been added. *Courtesy: I.W. County Records Office.*

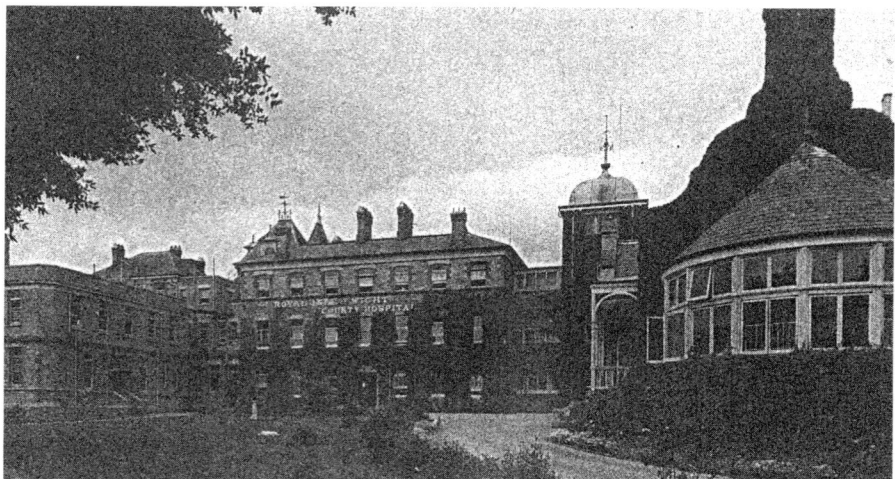

**Plate 4.** Royal Isle of Wight County Hospital. Ground and first floor wards have been built on (Cottle and Calthorpe wards). The word Infirmary has been removed. The domed tower on the right must be the Sanitary Tower designed by T.W. Cutler in 1902. *Courtesy: I.W. County Records Office.*

creation of a new Out-patient Department, with consulting rooms for physician and surgeon, a dispensary, a covered waiting porch and an Out-patient hall; above these were to be the new isolation wards for men and women with nurses' changing rooms and their duty room, and a bathroom with a mobile bath which could, it appears, be wheeled from one room to another; the buildings also included a new mortuary and a post-mortem room, a chapel of ease and a small room set aside for pathological investigations; this last was soon improved with the help of a donation from the Dowager Lady Calthorpe. The contract for this work went to Henry Curtis of Southampton and the cost was about £5,000 but of this, Mrs. Hathway of Quarrhurst gave the money for the Out-patient hall in memory of her husband who had been a member of the Committee for some years; and the cost of the fire escape was provided by Mrs. Pakenham-Mahon who later made other and larger gifts; the cost also was in part defrayed by the proceeds from the bazaar organised by Mr. and Mrs. Maybrick which raised £918.

The new buildings were opened in 1907 by Princess Beatrice.

The next addition was a new operating theatre together with an anaesthetic room, sterilising room and changing rooms for the nurses and doctors. Half the cost for this, £500, was available from an anonymous gift through Mr. A. Banks, one of the surgeons to the hospital at the time; and about £300 was derived from a memorial fund for the late Dr Groves; he had specified that this money was to go to the creation in particular of the sterilising and anaesthetic rooms.

A memorial to King Edward VII was to be the modernisation of the main block of the hospital or such portion of it as subscriptions might allow; but at first it was felt that a nurses' wing of 12 beds was needed and would be part of the eventual plan. It might be expected that the Great War would have put a close to any building during those years - 1914 to 1919; but a new Eye Ward, doubtless planned earlier was opened in 1914 - and was regarded as a memorial to King Edward VII; and about the same time an electric lift was installed and an X-ray room built on; the former was a gift from the Mayor and Mayoress of Ryde, and the X-ray apparatus given by Mrs. Dobie of Ryde, was said to be one of the best and most up-to-date in any provincial hospital.

Some years before this building the Committee seeking more accommodation had reviewed the use of the Milligan Convalescent Home. The fact was that it was substantially under-used and in 1909 plans were produced to restrict the convalescent accommodation to two double bedrooms on the upper floor together with sitting-rooms for men and ladies, and to use the lower floor to provide a committee room, a secretary's office, a nurses' sitting-room and dining-rooms and bedrooms for a Superintendent Nurse and for three maids. This allowed some re-arrangement in the centre block and gave rooms there for an Assistant House Surgeon, for the hall porter and a servants' dining room.

The Committee's objective now was to provide two large wards either by re-modelling of the centre block or by additional building; the first of these was named 'In loving memory of Captain R.H. Harington' by his widow in May 1915. He had been a member of the Committee; the ward was dedicated by the Bishop of Southampton on December 2nd 1915.

The next important addition was Wyndham Cottle Ward built in 1921-22 to the design of Mr. Oatley by Messrs Ball & Sons, the result of a legacy from Dr Wyndham Cottle who had been an honorary member of the consulting medical staff for some years. This ward was opened by Princess Beatrice on July 27th 1922. There is a note in the minutes that while this work was going on it, presumably, involved the closure of some staff bedrooms and five maids were lodged out in the London Hotel opposite the hospital at a charge of 5s each per week.

The two large wards on the ground floor were thus provided. Cottle Ward forming a wing which to some degree counterbalanced Victoria Ward on the other side. Until further building occurred this left a flat roof on top of Cottle Ward and here for a time a tent obtained from Messrs Selfridges was erected so that patients could lie out in it in favourable weather.

Further plans were now made for the reconstruction of the main part of the hospital in 1925. The first work was an enlargement of the kitchen which was carried out by Messrs Seely and Paget Architects; in 1928 a bigger reconstruction was planned and was to include six private wards in one block; a room for the medical staff; a second theatre for septic cases; a day room on each floor for the patients; and a small ward on each floor for noisy or very difficult cases; also a reception hall with a telephone box, and a separate room for electrotherapeutics and massage; and re-adaptation of the isolation wards. This planning involved some dispute in the committees. Stanley Hall, F.R.I.B.A. was the Architect first invited to submit a plan; but his first scheme costing about £50,000 was far beyond what the Committee could contemplate; he produced a modified plan costing about £15,000 but it seems that this involved converting Victoria Ward into an X-ray Department and building a new childrens' ward above Cottle Ward; and this plan was approved by the Building Committee and passed, but subsequently with representations from the Medical Committee the Chairman decided to disregard this vote and those plans were abandoned. This led to the resignation from the Building Committee of Miss Calthorpe and her brother, Admiral Calthorpe who felt that, as the original vote had been unanimous in favour of the plans, it was improper now to disregard it; the Chairman could only reply that he felt that he was acting in the interests of the hospital. The implication presumably was that the original decision had been hasty and made without full consideration. Both remained members of the General Committee and indeed rendered many future services to the hospital.

New plans were provided by Seely & Paget and were carried out involving an enlargement of the X-ray Department and a new ward over Cottle Ward, the funds for which had been obtained mainly by Miss Calthorpe who had collected £1,064 from the ladies of the Island and also £352 from Island children, made up of two miles of pennies; she had also obtained ten thousand bricks and ten tons of cement from a Mr. Saunders and two thousand bricks from the Carisbrooke Brick Company. The ward was named in recognition of her services and the furniture for the ward was provided by Admiral Calthorpe. Seely & Paget somehow managed to find rooms in the centre block for 12 nurses' bedrooms and for maids on the upper floor and they also remodelled the isolation ward. The new buildings were opened by Princess Beatrice on August 13th 1931.

This reconstruction must have also involved the formation of Elizabeth Ward, named for Princess Elizabeth, opposite Calthorpe Ward and approximately over Harington Ward. It was not until 1937 that, on the decision of the Medical Committee, the two wards on the ground floor, Harington and Cottle were designated as medical wards and the first floor pair, Calthorpe and Elizabeth as surgical. Meanwhile further buildings and reconstruction had created another ward on the second floor which was opened by Princess Beatrice also in 1937 and named after her. This ward being on the upper floor and close to the theatre was intended from the start for surgical patients and it came to be used exclusively for orthopaedic cases.

Two more important additions were to be built before the outbreak of war. A new Pathological Laboratory just inside the wall separating the grounds from Swanmore Road was built and opened in 1937 and of course this, after enlargement, remained the hospital laboratory right up to the time of the closure of the hospital.

The other important building was the King George V Nurses' Home in Adelaide Place built after much debate about costs by Messrs Rice of Brighton to the design of Seely & Paget at a cost of about £20,000, the land having been purchased for £1,600; the original estimate had been for £8,000 to £9,000 and when tenders for the first design were submitted they were between £22,000 and £24,000; this increase, - worthy perhaps of later times - caused the

Committee much concern and some members not surprisingly felt that they had been misled. The Building Committee with Sir Henry Sweetman in the chair in particular had discussions with the Architect and eventually a modified plan was accepted for some thousands of pounds less than the original. The opening of this home was planned for September 9th 1939 but was overtaken by events and the President was pleased to postpone the opening *sine die*; the house of course was already in use by then.

Up to this time the Out-patient and Casualty Departments had shared the same accommodation; this was becoming increasingly unsatisfactory and more so as the years went by so that two or three years before the war, there was talk of separating the two but nothing could be done at that time and the Committee had to temporise by re-arranging the available space and creating a small accessory theatre for dealing with surgical casualties; at one time the sister's office of the childrens' ward adjacent, or nearly so, to the Casualty Department was taken over for casualties and in 1942 a bedroom in the childrens' ward had to be refitted as an office for the almoner. At the other end of the hospital, earlier on, a temporary bathroom for resident nurses had been squeezed in under the main staircase, and by the end of the war more rooms in the convalescent home had been taken over for offices.

## Management

Lord Yarborough was the first President and after his death in 1862 Lord Heytesbury became President until 1891; he was succeeded by Prince Henry of Battenberg and after his death in 1896 Princess Beatrice, Princess Henry of Battenberg, succeeded him as the Governor of the Island and President of the hospital until her own death in 1944.

The Committee of Management continued its weekly meetings right up until 1930. It must have been the organisation which ran the hospital although of course it made its annual report to the Governors who had their say at the Annual General Meeting and at occasional special meetings requested by the Committee. The Governors also elected members to the Committee; after a time however the Committee members and Vice Presidents came to include the Mayors of Ryde and Newport, the Arch-Deacon of the Island, the Chairman of the County Council after 1890, and the Member of Parliament. Very often retired honorary medical officers were also appointed to the Committee.

The early statutes mentioned that all complaints were to be referred to the

Committee - an attitude which might be approved nowadays, but it is doubtful whether the manner of dealing with the complaints, in some cases at least, would have found favour in modern eyes; in 1875, it was reported that a Mrs. Maynard had remarked in the presence of two patients that it was a pity that patients were discharged before they were cured. A motion was carried in the Committee, unanimously, that Mrs. Maynard be not allowed to enter the Infirmary for any purpose; a copy to be sent to Mrs. Maynard. Later she offered an explanation of her remark (the explanation is not quoted), but the Committee regretted that in the interest of the institution, they adhered to their resolution. After further exchange, she explained that all she had done was to tell a patient who was about to discharge himself against advice that it was a great pity that he should go out before he was cured. However, there was no further action!

In 1881 the British Medical Association held its annual conference in Ryde under the Presidency of Benjamin Barrow formerly a Honorary Surgeon and now a member of the Committee and recently Mayor of Ryde; during this time, August 13th to 18th, the Infirmary and Convalescent Home were opened to members of the B.M.A. on presentation of their cards.

In 1889 Queen Victoria visited the hospital accompanied by her oldest daughter, the Dowager Empress of Germany, Prince Henry of Battenberg and the Princesses Sophia and Margarethe of Prussia. After this visit, the Queen sent the hospital seven framed pictures commemorating it; one wonders what has become of them. It was also after this visit that at the Queen's wish the name was changed to the Royal Isle of Wight Infirmary and County Hospital; it was in 1906 that it was decreed the title should no longer include the word infirmary.

The introduction of the Convalescent Home in 1878 had required new regulations. The home was to have a lady Superintendent who later served as Assistant Matron to the hospital and stood in for the Matron during holidays. The House Surgeon was in medical charge and was authorised to decide the diet and presumably any medication of each inmate; the Medical Committee considered that he should attend inmates, and because of the extra work imposed upon him, he should be paid not less that £20 a year out of the accounts of the home. Persons with pulmonary consumption or other disease in advanced state; those requiring medical and nursing treatment; those of unsound mind or liable to fits; or recovering from contagious disease; or who had not been vaccinated, should, according to the Medical Committee, be excluded; also those under eight years of age and those in an advanced state of pregnancy. These recommendations were accepted by the Committee save that they did not exclude those in an advance state of pregnancy; also they decided not to raise the House Surgeon's salary deeming that his work would not be increased; later it was decreed that the House Surgeon need not visit the home daily but need only come in response to a call and that he should consult with the appropriate honorary staff whenever necessary.

There was, I think, never a chapel in the hospital but services were held in the Infirmary and from time to time a room was set aside for the use of the Chaplain; in 1886 there was a minute that a patient had been admonished by the Chairman for failing to attend divine service. In that same year the Committee appointed four ladies to visit the hospital; they should go round the wards and talk to the patients but should not read to them or pray with them. The Committee did have to restrain the activities of the Gospel Readers who were excessively persistent in their efforts to preach to the patients. In 1886 also the Committee decided that for the first time the buildings and contents should be insured, - the main building for £2,400, the fever wards for £400, and the lodge for £160; the contents of these three components for £600, £100 and £40 respectively.

There was continuing difficulty in accommodating nurses and in 1888 the use of a small ward for a nurses' bedroom was debated; an alternative was to employ nurses from a nursing institute in George Street, Ryde; it was thought better and cheaper to accommodate their own nurses in the hospital.

As mentioned earlier it seems that from the start the House Surgeon visited patients in their homes; presumably, these visits were limited to Ryde and its immediate environs. Now it was understood that visits were to cease; this supposed decision provoked a very vigorous protest from the Clergy of the Island who asserted that the 'Custom of visiting out-patients unable to attend the hospital is in the nature of a contract since congregations subscribe to the hospital; and it has been an accepted custom since the foundation'. The Committee agreed to receive a deputation of Clergy to consider the matter and they assured the deputation that the House Surgeon would continue to visit old patients when directed by the honorary staff to do so; it seems that those who were elderly and those that were too ill to attend as out-patients benefitted from this service. I have found no indication when these visits to out-patients ceased; the work within the hospital was steadily increasing in all directions, the numbers of beds and bed occupancy, the operations, the attendance of out-patients and the numbers of casualties all rose from year to year; the House Surgeon must have been a very busy man and one supposes that the visits gradually declined; certainly they cannot have been continued after the introduction of Lloyd George's National Insurance Act of 1912.

The rules of the hospital were revised about the turn of the century; I have not been able to find any copy of these revised rules but a later revision in 1930 implies that for the most part they were then left unchanged. Among other arrangements there was to be an election committee for the appointment of honorary medical staff, composed of the acting honorary medical staff, the elected members of the General Committee and up to ten Governors. The House Surgeon was not to be entitled to a holiday unless he was re-appointed after a year's work; if absent for any other reason he must himself appoint a locum tenens acceptable to the honorary staff, at his own expense; it is fair to add that long before 1930 more generous arrangements were sometimes made for holidays. Honorary surgeons were to retire at the age of 60; other doctors at the age of 65. There was a further entry about the duties of the House Surgeon in 1920; he or she must be present at all operations; in the absence of a pathologist he must keep the post-mortem room in good order and must order or make the necessary post-mortem examinations; he must keep an inventory of all instruments and keep the medical notes in safe custody and in such a way that they could be readily available when required; he must never leave the hospital before 1 p.m. Some years prior to this entry the House Surgeon had given a course of lectures to nurses; he or she had to inform the Committee of these lectures and he was paid £10 for the course. Later, lectures were taken over by the honorary medical staff and the care of patients' notes was passed on to the ward sisters. The Committee might refuse admission for a patient and it might order a patient to be discharged unless the medical staff requested otherwise. The list of patients now excluded was simplified; the insane, epileptics, and those who would not benefit were not to be admitted; clearly this left the matter in the hands of the medical staff.

The door to the Out-patient Department was to be open from 7 a.m. to 7 p.m. An assistant House Surgeon was first appointed at a salary of £60 per annum in 1909; he or she was required to be competent as an anaesthetist and at X-ray work; regrettably the House Surgeon and the first Assistant H.S. working together did not get on well, and after the House Surgeon failed to attend at an operation, where he was required, he was asked to leave; the assistant also left without completing his term and no further appointment of an assistant was made until very much later, in the 1930s. Advertisements after this time usually specified that candidates for the post of H.S. should be competent anaesthetists and at X-ray work!

There were some less serious matters to be considered; the Secretary of the Royal National Hospital, Mr. de Vine, sought the Committee's co-operation in amateur theatricals, - the profits to be shared; this was agreed. The nurses suggested that a tennis court might be provided in the grounds of the convalescent home; this could not be managed, but the Chairman presented the nurses with a badminton set. The Committee joined with the British Hospital Association in asking the Post Master General to provide a free telephone service for hospitals; they also sought freedom from legacy duty. (No marks for guessing the answer to these requests). In 1923 the Committee offered to pay the annual subscription of 8s-6d for any nurses who wished to join the Ryde Sports Club, 15 of them did so.

About 1918 the conversion of the convalescent home into a nurses' home was suggested, - some rooms were still urgently needed, and by 1923 with an increase in the number of probationer nurses this was brought about.

When the use of wireless in hospital was first discussed, it was decided that it should on no account be installed; this was in 1924, but within that year the *County Press* had offered a set free for the use of patients and by 1926 wireless for patients was conceded; headphones were to be used except in the childrens' ward. In 1932 wireless was available in all wards and Col. Murray, a Committee member, was asked to supervise the hospital wireless installation and service.

Lady life Governors were asked in 1921 to set up a committee to assist in organising working parties, entertainments, collections and fund-raising. A needlework group was established mainly by Miss Calthorpe, and over several years made large contributions to the hospital producing over two thousand articles in four years.

In 1925 the medical staff recommended that no smoking should be allowed in the hospital except at Christmas; this recommendation was repeated a few years later; in 1933 however it was agreed that limited smoking, namely from 1.00 to 1.45 p.m. and between 7.00 and 8.00 p.m. would be allowed; the ward sister had authority to disallow it if necessary and she was to keep a supply of tobacco under lock and key.

Out-patients and their accompanying supporters sometimes then, as later, had long waits in the Out-patient Department; the Committee found in 1925 that it could not supply refreshments but it authorised those waiting to bring food with them; in 1932 the womens' section of Toc H offered to provide a canteen, but it seems that soon after that, a local catering firm took over the service.

The special departments began to appear early in the century. The X-ray Department, the Ear, Nose and Throat Department and Eye Department about 1904; a Venereal Disease Clinic came in 1917, and Orthopaedic and Genito-Urinary Clinics in 1930. In 1912 the comment was made that the National Insurance Act meant that a large class of patients, hitherto unable to pay for treatment at home, and thus obliged to come for treatment to the hospital, would now be entitled to treatment and consultation at home. This, it was thought, might necessitate new regulations about admissions and treatment but I can find no record of any such rules and admission by letter of recommendation continued for more than twenty years to come.

In 1914 a motor ambulance was provided. Before this, from 1885 a spring van had been available for patients too ill to come otherwise; the cost of the horse and the driver at that time had to be defrayed by the patient or a friend. No charge was made for the motor ambulance when it was introduced but those who could afford it, or who had friends who could afford it, were expected to contribute.

In 1926 there was a visit from the Prince of Wales on his way to Ventnor to open the Lampard-Green Nurses' Home at the R.N.H.; during which he made a presentation to the retiring Chairman, Mr. Blair Cochrane.

In December 1926 a surprising minute was written when the Chairman ruled - in reply to an enquiry by Mr. (later Sir Henry) Sweetman, 'Since patients were admitted with the approval of the Committee, members had the right to make enquiries as to the nature of the disease specified on the medical certificate of the letter of recommendation'.

This ruling seems to indicate, if taken literally, that any or all of the Committee had the right to be informed of the diagnosis of any or all of the patients admitted. I find it difficult to believe that this was what was intended, and I feel no doubt that the medical staff, - both resident and honorary visiting - would have explained to any committee member who sought information the nature of confidence. It is well known of course that the diagnosis in many patients on admission is known to their friends, their families and sometimes indeed the public, but to have the right to demand the information on the medical certificate is a different matter; what led to or what was behind the original enquiry one can only speculate.

The following year the Chairman reported that he had been invited to take part in the management of an institution formerly known as the childrens' hostel, - now apparently called Ryde Hospital or possibly Ryde Hospital for Women and Children. He told the Committee he had replied that he regretted he could not recognise any hospital other than the Royal County Hospital although he was in sympathy with the idea of a childrens' hostel.

This 'Hostel for Ailing Children' was established at Southlands in Park Road and was active between 1921 - 1929 superintended by Miss Friend, it seems that it was supported largely by a grant from the Ministry of Health; that patients came from all parts of England; that the hospital would accept chronic cases unsuitable for a general hospital, and that there was a charge of 12s-6d a week; Lady Simeon had been interested in it and had sought the co-operation of the County Hospital. In February 1929 a letter came from the childrens' hospital; its committee had found themselves unable to maintain it and offered the County Hospital two hundred guineas to take it over. A sub committee was appointed to consider this offer but were unable to recommend it and it was declined.

It has been mentioned that weekly committee meetings continued right up to 1930. It was then that a House Committee was formed which was to meet weekly and the General Management Committee met thereafter just once a month. The House Committee received notice of such things as admissions and discharges of the week and they dealt with appointments of domestic staff, minor repairs or requisitions, etc.; often the meeting was attended only by two or three members; the monthly committee meetings continued to deal with the main running of the hospital and as before any major items of building, expenditure, etc. were referred to the Annual General Meeting of Governors.

At a meeting on December 30th 1930 it was commented that H.R.H. Princess Beatrice, the President had not visited the hospital for some time, and it was said that she was somewhat out of sympathy with the hospital because they had not undertaken training for V.A.D. nurses; it was now agreed that such training should be introduced and the President opened the new buildings in 1931.

It was not until the time of the Second World War that a trained or qualified almoner was appointed; but in 1923 a Mr. A. Wilson, who had been appointed as a collector some time before, took on the role of almoner and was asked to carry on in accordance with the instructions used at Portsmouth Royal Hospital; he received at first a salary of £70 but this was increased later up to £200 yearly; among his activities, with the blessing of the Committee, he organised an all Island annual whist championship which for many years made a useful and quite considerable contribution of a few hundred pounds each year to the hospital funds.

It was in 1937 after the new Beatrice Ward had been opened by the President with the relief of congestion in the male wards that the medical and surgical wards were separated. The wards on the ground floor were hereafter medical and those on the first and second floor surgical - including the ophthalmic and orthopaedic wards.

It was in this year also that a second House Surgeon was finally added to the establishment; his salary was £130 yearly, the H.S. at this time having £200 a year; and in 1939 just before the war, the second House Surgeon was 'converted' into a House Physician, and so things remained for many years.

On August 30th 1939 several patients were discharged in order that some beds should be available for anticipated casualties in the presumptive crisis. This was criticised in the Committee, but Dr Stratton, speaking presumably on behalf of all the honorary medical officers, said that it had been considered that an emergency was already there, and he had decided and acted to the best of his ability; those who remember the times may feel that he was justified; evacuees were already coming across from Portsmouth and sand bags were being filled; however at that time, there as elsewhere, there was no flood of casualties and by mid September the hospital was full again.

With the onset of war of course the hospital became part of the Emergency Medical Service as did all others, but it does not seem to have made very much immediate difference to the running of the hospital. Shortages of staff - domestic staff, nursing staff and doctors were of course a problem there during the war.

In 1942, Ryde House was taken over by agreement for the use of patients suitable for transfer from the hospital, or possibly by direct admission; the medical staff, Dr Dockray in particular, thought this preferable to the possibility of Island patients having to be moved to some more or less distant place on the mainland. However, Ryde House was not in use for very long, - being closed in 1944; but in that year also Mr. G.R. Brigstocke offered the hospital the use of St. Vincent's Home as a convalescent home for the hospital, in memory of his two sons. This offer was accepted. However, as things turned out the hospital did not find a use for a convalescent home of this type; there was a suggestion that it should be used for staff accommodation but this was not in accordance with the terms on which it had been offered and by agreement in 1947 the association was discontinued; St. Vincent's of course subsequently came a residential home for ex-service men.

Maintenance and standards must have been difficult during the war and in February 1945 it was reported that the childrens' ward was unfit to receive patients, and Dr Fairley, the County Medical Officer, was asked to arrange for children to be admitted to Scio House in Shanklin until Victoria Ward could be made ready again.

About this time, Mr. Gordon who had served the hospital as Secretary for 45 years was due to resign; he was given a part-time nominal appointment as Honorary Supervisor of Accounts to enable him to complete 50 years of service.

The committee meeting on August 15th 1945, V.J. Day, faced plenty of problems. Catering costs were rising steeply and there was some dissatisfaction with food and feeding; a new kitchen superintendent was appointed and produced an improved service but she left to go abroad after only about one year; extensive re-planning and re-equipment of the kitchen was discussed in 1947; it is worth mentioning that, at this time, pig-swill was still collected from the kitchen and sold locally, the contract being worth £60 a year. Accommodation for both patients, nurses and domestic staff was a continuing problem and the difficulty of obtaining equipment and materials compounded it in those early years, as will be well remembered by those who can recall the times of austerity. Elizabeth and Mary and Cottle Wards all needed extensive repair and re-fitting; work was needed to provide a better Out-patient Department and to improve the casualty arrangements.

During these years also the decision was taken to abandon the internal laundry and a contract was made with the Vectis Laundry and was considered to be no more expensive than re-equipping the hospital laundry would have been.

Having filled all the available space on its original site, the hospital now looked for houses in nearby Partlands Avenue. The first house to be taken on lease, the Towers, served as a preliminary training school for nurses and provided at first accommodation for nine student nurses and for a sister tutor, assistant matron and two domestic workers.

The Victor Nursing home at that time occupying some houses in Partlands Avenue was considered for private accommodation; however this did not come about and it was now that the private wards were established in what had formerly been the isolation block overlying the Casualty Department; the Chairman, Aubrey Wickham died in 1947 and the refurbished wing providing seven, or ultimately nine single wards, was named in his memory the Aubrey Wickham wing. Some of the domestic staff were again housed in the London Inn and two ward sisters were allowed to live out receiving an allowance of £100 a year for this.

## Staff

The sources of information - chiefly the minutes of weekly, monthly or annual meetings of committees and Governors do not give much detail of the nursing staff and the servants who keep all hospitals running. However, they did receive some consideration and at the very start in 1849, a week's diet allowance was set down for the servants, all of whom were of course resident.

They were to have:-

| | |
|---|---|
| Bread and flour | 1 gallon |
| Beer | 7 pints |
| Butter | 1/2 lb. |
| Sugar | 1/2 lb. |
| Cheese | 1/2 lb. |
| Meat | 7 lb. |
| Tea | 2 1/2 oz. |
| Milk | 2 1/2 pints |
| Vegetables | twice daily |

So foodwise they did not do so badly. The Matron was in charge of the nursing staff, but there is little to be found about their numbers although there is mention from time to time of appointments, resignations and occasional dismissals. In 1875, the accounts show that five nurses received £4.10s each quarter, £18 a year; at this stage, the Matron whose salary had varied between £10 and £30 yearly was up to £40 a year and the H.S. £50; house maids had £3 a quarter, laundress £3.10s, and cook £5.

By 1881, there were five nurses and two house maids; the complement of patients would then have been about 30 plus 10 for the fever beds; extra nurses were appointed when there were epidemics. By 1885, the total expenditure on servants wages was £305.10s in the year; the 'servants' perhaps included house maids, porters, a dispenser (who was also a porter) and nurses. The dispenser at that time had 25s a week - £65 a year; if the remaining staff had an average wage of £20 a year, this would allow about a dozen staff of all categories.

Nurses in those early days of course had no particular training, though presumably they received some instructions from the Matron. In 1863 there was a note that no nurse had been available to attend to a man admitted in the night with a fractured skull; the House Surgeon was instructed to ensure that the Matron was always informed of such admissions.

The career of one hospital servant, George Dash, was so remarkable as surely to merit a paragraph. He was born in London in 1824; both his parents died before he was thirteen and in 1837 he came to Newport to live with his uncle. Soon after this, he joined the Royal Navy, but was invalided out in 1845. He was appointed as gardener and porter to the hospital before it opened in 1847-48 and among his duties in the early years, he pumped up the water from the well near the front gate to the tank in the roof twice daily; this heavy work, it was said, led to a marked muscular development and he was accustomed to carrying patients whenever necessary. In 1858 he was given permission to marry provided that he lived in the lodge which was built for him. In 1860 a bell was fixed to ring in his home from the main door or gate at night, - so his job included that of night porter. In 1867, the Chairman informed his Committee that the porter (George Dash) was in the habit of extracting teeth and dressing wounds in the absence of the House Surgeon. The Committee resolved that he should not act in this capacity except in the presence of the House Surgeon, and in 1873, he was prohibited altogether from these functions. The problem of dental extraction was partly solved, when the Chairman informed the Committee that he had had a letter from a Mr. Harington 'Declaring his willingness to extract all the teeth sent to him by the Infirmary'.

Later George Dash took on the job of dispenser, and it was at his suggestion that the dispenser's salary was increased to £65 a year; later again the Committee decided that the House Surgeon was the man who had legal responsibility for running the dispensary. In 1898, the minutes state that 'George Dash, an old and respected servant of the hospital, was to act in future only as general porter and not as dispenser.' A lady was appointed to be Dispenser and Secretary and clearly George Dash had been doing the job for about 15 years. By 1900 he had more or less given up regular work but he lived in the lodge with his wife and was always pleased to help any of the staff in any way he could and he kept the front of the hospital tidy. He had three married daughters and in 1919 was a widower. He finally retired and left his lodge which was then taken over to provide nursing accommodation. He went to live with one of his three married daughters in Carisbrooke having served the hospital for over 70 years. He died in 1923 and was buried in Ryde Cemetery. Through his executor and eldest son-in-law the hospital received a bequest of £25 from him.

By the end of the century, nursing had become a profession and nurse training something of a reality. In 1888 on the initiative of one of the Honorary Medical Officers of the day - Dr Davey - a course of lectures for nurses was started, and in the same year the Matron was authorised to choose nurses' uniform dresses; much later in 1920, the Committee minuted the need to increase the number of probationers (as student nurses were then called) from 16 to 20, since the hospital had become a recognised training school for nurses, - in order to give nurses 'the requisite time for study so that they might pass the rather difficult examinations which were necessary to increase the staff'; later again the Committee decided to offer six prizes for nurses who achieved examinational success.

In January 1889 a nurse wished to leave the service of the hospital because she could earn more, £25 a year, in private work than she got at the hospital, - £22 a year; she was told to go and get it. In 1890 it was agreed that the Honorary Medical Officers might 'borrow' a nurse from the hospital for private nursing, if and so long as she was not needed in the hospital; she was to return on the Matron's request and was to be paid for her private work by the Medical Officer.

In March 1892 the Committee purchased a book of tickets for ozone baths for the use of the nursing staff!

The services of trained nurses outside the hospital, i.e. in the district and the community were becoming called for, and a motion was carried that 'The Isle of Wight should provide trained nurses in the community and a building should be put up for the purpose (presumably for training nurses and perhaps for administering the service) but the hospital funds should not be used for this purpose'.

The nurses were hard pressed in those days at times; in 1908 there were two children in the infectious diseases ward with Scarlet Fever; the nurse looking after them had no time off day or night; the Matron, asked for help, sent a maid who had recently had Scarlet Fever.

After the X-ray Department came into use the radiographer was under the supervision of the Matron, and the Matron herself, at her own request, was authorised to receive instruction in radiography and to travel to London for the purpose.

A night sister (Miss C. Elgar) was appointed in 1911 at a salary of £28 a year. Nurses were difficult to recruit in the years before the First World War; and the probationers' salary which had been at £8 a year was raised to £12 for the second year and £18 for the third year; this shortage being the case, it was perhaps rather surprising that the Committee refused to allow Lady Baird's Red Cross nurses to attend on the wards; a further request for this was rejected by the Medical Officers in 1913; however by 1915 it was agreed that the Red Cross nurses working in nearby Haslewood should come for instruction and to help in the ward work, four at a time, and under the orders of the Matron. In 1918 a shortage of nurses called for closure of Harington Ward and the private wards temporarily and this recurred the next winter; but a round robin from the probationer nurses asking the Committee for a rise in salary was rejected, - they were told that such applications might come only through the Matron.

The House Surgeon usually, as now, held his appointment for six months or a year and right up until the end of the century he functioned also as Secretary. His secretarial duties ended in 1898 when the newly appointed dispenser also took over secretarial duties; save that he still had to attend the

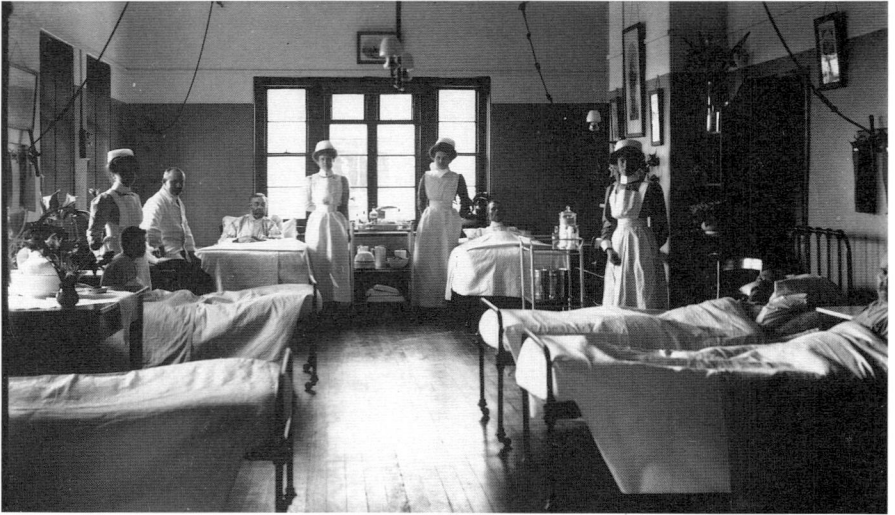

**Plate 5**. Interior view of a ward: the dresses suggest that this photo was taken early this century. *Courtesy: Roy Brinton*.

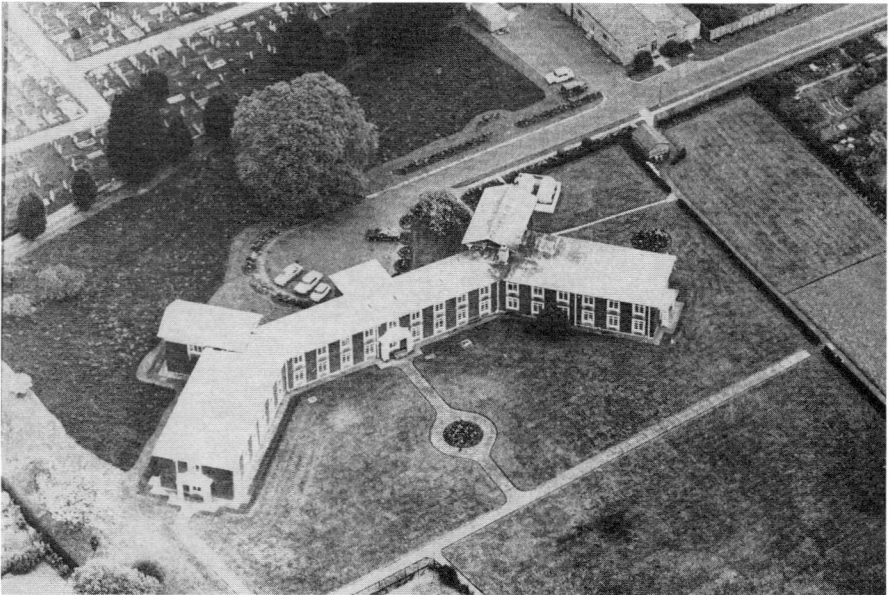

**Plate 6**. King George V Nurses' Home - Royal County Hospital. *Courtesy: Mr. J. Lewis (& others?)*.

committee meetings and keep the minute book; in 1896 the medical staff had complained that the House Surgeon had to spend too much time in his secretarial work. I think that with the appointment of a full-time secretary he finally ceased to have any duties in that respect.

The Honorary Medical Staff of course gave their services; and as the hospital increased in size and numbers of beds the work must have taken up an increasing amount of their time; in return they were presumably entitled to treat their private patients in the few beds reserved for such paying patients. These were never numerous and right up to the time of the Health Service, and indeed so long after that as the hospital provided any private beds, it was always accepted that any emergency case could, if necessary, be admitted to one of the private beds. In 1878 Dr Broom-Pinniger was granted the use of a room in the hospital for the annual meeting of the Isle of Wight Medico-Chirurgical Society. The Honorary Medical Officers were mostly doctors practising in Ryde, although certainly several came from other parts of the Island; at the very start Mr. Bloxam came from Newport and Dr Martin from Ventnor; and later certainly Dr Waterworth and Dr Stratton of Newport were among the staff.

I should mention here Dr A. Wade a House Surgeon who remained in post throughout the First World War; junior staff residents were difficult to come by at that time, and the Committee recorded their gratitude to him for staying on. Another House Surgeon who became a senior member of the staff was Dr Horsbrugh who took on the job of Honorary Pathologist for a time before he was followed by Dr Firman-Edwards in 1921. He, Dr Horsbrugh, had the golfing distinction of having done the longest ever hole in two, at the fifteenth hole at Manchester, - 504 yards! I do not know whether this is still a record.

I have already referred to the earliest record of dental work in the hospital; in November 1878, the name of the Dental Surgeon to the hospital - Mr. Canter - was included in the list of Honorary Medical Staff and soon after the turn of the century there were two dentists on the staff, one slightly confusingly, was a Mr. W.G. Daish; the second one was Mr. W. Griffin who was appointed to the post in 1903 and after the retirement of Mr. Daish he carried on alone; he served the hospital for 30 years retiring in 1933; in retirement he was a famous gardener and walker and lived to be 100.

At the very beginning there was reference to a laboratory but there was no indication of any pathological work until after the turn of the century at which time the new buildings designed by T.W. Cutler included a pathological laboratory; this was renovated or improved and equipped with the help of the Dowager Lady Calthorpe as already indicated. In 1913 new equipment was available and some sort of pathological service could be offered not merely to the hospital but to doctors on the Island; and a list of investigations was issued:-

| | |
|---|---|
| Identification of organisms other than Tubercle Bacilli | 2/- |
| Examination of Sputum | 2/- |
| Blood Count | 3/- |
| Widal reaction | 2/6d |
| Throat swab | 2/- |
| Cutting and mounting specimens | 5/- to 6/- |
| Examination of urine | 2/6d |

Dr Firman-Edwards continued as Honorary Pathologist until 1938, - though in the meantime he had also been for a while Medical Officer of Health for Ryde and in 1937 together with John Dockray he became an Honorary Physician. By 1938 pathology investigations had become more frequent and numerous and a more extensive service was needed. At this juncture, Dr Thornton and Dr Darmady, Pathologists at Salisbury offered to undertake the work and to visit regularly provided that a new laboratory was built; this was done, - the low building close to the Swanmore Road entrance was put up for £800 and after additions and alterations served this purpose up to the time of the closure of the hospital. One of the two Honorary Pathologists visited the hospital regularly each week and it was agreed that they would give their services but would undertake work privately referred to them by doctors on the Island; a trained technician, or later several technicians, worked in the laboratory and the service continued through the war; soon after the end of the war Dr Thornton retired when new arrangements were made at the start of the National Health Service.

The medical officers in 1928 asked for the appointment of a salaried part-time anaesthetist and Dr Agnes Bryce-Smith was appointed and served the hospital for two years; after that it was decided that the anaesthetists should be members of the honorary medical staff and appointments were made from 1931; while preparing this book I had the opportunity of speaking to Dr Sutherland who died in 1993; she told me that she was the first honorary anaesthetist to be appointed, in 1933, but according to the minutes there were others before her including Dr Collie who retired from the job in 1931; Mr. O'Donoghue and Mr. Liesching both worked as honorary anaesthetists for a period. Dr Sutherland continued in the services of the hospital until 1945 and after that in general practice until 1959.

In the years between the wars, many of the House Surgeons were lady doctors and several of them were re-appointed for a second or even a third spell and received the approbation of the Committee. In 1927 it was minuted that Dr Bonhote, a lady doctor, had given a blood transfusion to a young patient and was considered to have saved his life thereby and the Committee recorded their appreciation. The implication was that she had given a transfusion of her own blood. After that the medical officers recommended that a list of donors should be prepared and later the Red Cross Service took over the administration of blood transfusion, until later again it was organised from Portsmouth.

The first X-ray Department was opened in 1904 and a new X-ray room was built shortly before the First World War. The radiographer at that time had a salary of £40 a year and was, as mentioned, under the supervision of the Matron. In 1913 diagnostic X-rays were recorded in 96 cases; 'high frequency treatment' was given to 139 patients. Dr Burrell was the first radiologist to be appointed. In 1936 a new department for radium treatment was opened and was served by a visiting consultant who came monthly from Southampton.

An Ophthalmic service was recommended in 1896 and a clinic was opened soon after that. Mr. May was the first eye surgeon appointed to the hospital early in the century. An Ear, Nose and Throat Department started in 1922; Dr Stuart was the first visiting ENT surgeon.

Infectious diseases were, especially up to the time in the 1890s when infectious diseases hospitals came into being, a continuing preoccupation of the medical officers. Cholera, Smallpox and Scarlet Fever were ones most frequently mentioned and all hospitals tried to avoid ever dealing with Smallpox. Before the hospital was opened there was an epidemic of Cholera in Newport and an offer was made for the use of the hospital wards for patients from Newport and was gratefully accepted by the Board of Guardians who offered to furnish presumably temporary wards that were needed; however I could find no evidence that this offer was actually taken up. In 1866 the medical officers at the request of the Committee presented recommendations for action in case of an epidemic of cholera:-

1. All available beds to be appropriated (presumably this implied that other admissions should be postponed sine die).
2. Patients to be kept separate and to have separate attendants.
3. The cheapest available bedding to be used so that it could be destroyed after use.

A few years later in 1870 the medical officers were urging better accommodation for fevers and stressing the need for the nurses and the laundry to be kept separate; the Sanitary Committee of the Ryde Borough Council was involved in the provision of accommodation for infectious diseases and apparently agreed to pay part of the expenses of the patients. In May of 1871 this Sanitary Committee apparently sought permission to build a temporary hospital in the grounds of the Ryde Infirmary; this was declined, - it seems that it was to be used for Smallpox. During that decade also, there was some dispute between the Ryde Borough Council and the hospital about admission of patients with Scarlet Fever and some exchanges between the Ryde Medical Officer of Health and the Hospital Committee and medical officers; it appears that there was at that time a borough hospital to which at least some patients with infectious diseases would be admitted; although the Ryde Isolation Hospital, off Rosemary Lane, was certainly not built until late in the 1880s.

It is appropriate to mention here, that in 1873 Mr. B. Barrow finally resigned. He had been a medical officer since the opening of the hospital twenty-four years earlier. His resignation was accepted 'With great regret and a deep sense of obligation', and in March 1874 he accepted the post of Honorary Consulting Surgeon; his criticisms did not end with that. He became a member of the Committee and in 1875 he was complaining of the filthy state of the wards, lobbies, sculleries and Out-patient Department. He went on to become the Mayor of Ryde and in 1881 President of the British Medical Association, as already mentioned.

Debate about the use of the fever wards continued; they were, one supposes, often empty and it was obviously tempting to use them for much needed staff accommodation or later to house the patients from the general wards when they were over-filled; in 1893 the Committee wished to close the fever wards, and it was specified that cases of Cholera should not be admitted; the closed wards were re-opened in 1894 and doctors were notified that a charge of one guinea weekly would be made for domestic patients. The next year, a minute in July said that there was no accommodation available in either the general or fever wards. Finally in 1907 or possibly earlier, it was decreed that the isolation wards were intended only for hospital in-patients who happened to develop infectious fevers while in hospital. By that time of course there were isolation hospitals available in Ryde, Sandown and Shanklin, and Ventnor; when new demands imposed further strain upon the accommodation in 1914, it was specified that infectious cases arising in the hospital might be transferred to the isolation hospital at Smallbrook, the County Hospital would in that case pay something for the use of the beds.

Medical staff and nurses were not the only ones who were at times busy and hard pressed. In 1926 à propos of the need for upgrading or renewal of the kitchen, it was noted that one cook and one maid had to provide six staff breakfasts between 7 a.m. and 9 a.m. (patients' breakfasts were cooked by the night nurses); nurses' dinners; dinner for the maids and for the House Surgeon; hot dinners at night for the Matron, House Surgeon, night nurses and paying patients; supper for the nurses and servants; all this, in addition presumably, to the regular dinners and suppers for the patients.

## Finances

Finding enough money to keep the hospital running and to enlarge and improve it as seen desirable or necessary was from the start a persistent problem. In the hospital's whole independent life of 99 years, there was only just one spell of a few years when income exceeded expenditure. The hospital had not been going very long before a committee or sub-committee was formed to consider means of economising.

In the very early years collectors were appointed in the principle towns on the Island: unpaid but authorised to keep 10% of what they collected. Also, when servants, male or female, were admitted, their employers were expected to pay, 1/6d daily.

The quarterly expenditure between 1852 and 1865 naturally varied, but it generally kept at around an average figure of £230 ± £30; in 1865 it rose to £274; thus in the first ten years or so the expenses were kept within £1,000 p.a. In 1875, with the increase in beds, it had gone up to £450 a quarter. During these years and for some time afterwards the accounts as presented included a House Surgeon's account and a Matron's account. The former dealt with instruments and thermometers; drugs; wines and spirits; stationery; printing; disinfecting apparatus; incidentals; and, rather surprisingly, tithes; it is perhaps surprising also to find that wines and spirits under this heading constituted often up to 10% of the House Surgeon's account; malt liquors appeared in the general account for provisions and were presumably regarded as part of the regular food, perhaps for servants rather than patients, while wines and spirits were regarded as medicinal. Altogether in the first quarter of 1875 the House Surgeon's account came to £45-11s. The Matron's incidentals came to £26-6s; salaries were:-

| | | | |
|---|---|---|---|
| H.S. | - £12-10-0 | Five Nurses, each at - | £4-10-0 |
| Matron | - £10 - 0-0 | A house maid | - £3 - 0-0 |
| Dispenser | - 11 guineas | Laundress | - £3-10-0 |

In the way of food, meat for the quarter cost £97-16; ale and porter - £19-13; milk and eggs - £26-17; potatoes and vegetables - £8-13; groceries - £46; fish and essence of meat - £3-14. In some years there is a heading for bread and flour, but not in this particular one. Presumably it is included in groceries. Coal and wood came to £30; gas - £13-13; the chimney sweep - £4-6; and incidentals £2-12; general expenses including payments to the painter, decorator, draper, iron-monger, upholsterer and builder - £29. Electricity of course would not yet have been installed, and the entry for the sweep reminds us that all the wards as well as staff rooms, etc. must have been heated by coal and wood.

Major Leeds, the Chairman commented in 1880 that after 30 years the endowment funds of the hospital were only £10,000; by 1888, including £5,500 from Miss Milligan for the convalescent home, they had reached £23,842. In 1890 the Treasurer was in difficulties; a street collection, presumably a forerunner of the hospital flag day, produced £166; in 1894 a Samaritan fund was initiated to provide artificial limbs and other surgical appliances. In 1900, 25 years after the previous figures, the total expenditure was £4,163; provisions cost £1,324; surgery and dispensary £398 (of which £41 was on wines and spirits); domestic £470 including coal £197 and gas £135; establishment charge £132; rent £28-15; salaries (including the HS and his locum and some petty cash payments) £78; Matron £45; sub matron £20; nurses collectively £210; extra nurses £82; servants £29; the Secretary £37-10; and the Chaplain £30.

Income this year came from:-
annual subscriptions - £840; donations - £227; Hospital Sunday Association - £29; work people's contributions - £159; congregational collections - £111; entertainments - £86; miscellaneous - £11. Investments yielded £10; interest on deposits - £9; and the sale of dripping and waste paper - £3-14. Ordinary income was £2,825-13; extraordinary legacies of £1,824 brought the total up to £4,650. Gifts mentioned this year included games and toys; linen; clothes and bedding; books and journals; the harvest festival - flowers, fruit and eggs; also framed pictures; a box of cigars; linoleum for the hall and stairs and teak for flooring. In this year there were 474 in-patients; 1360 out-patients; 195 operations; there were 78 residents in the convalescent home.

By 1913, the year immediately before the First World War there was urgent need for more income; of course during the war as would be expected expenditure increased and each year the gap between income and expenses rose. It was commented in 1919 that it was impossible to maintain the hospital on less than £6,000 yearly - ten years earlier £3,600 had sufficed; renewals and repairs needed had accumulated during the war; by 1920 the excess of expenditure over income reached nearly £2,000 and it was feared that the voluntary system might soon come to an end; in 1920 there was an appeal for wage earners to increase their contributions; it was mentioned that many patients had been glad to make donations.

In 1925, regulations for private patients were issued; the charge was 4 guineas weekly for a shared ward, 6 guineas for a single ward; the accommodation was available for Isle of Wight residents requiring surgery; rooms could not be reserved more than 36 hours before admission; patients must conform to the ordinary hospital rules; emergency admissions could seek advice from outside specialists with the consent of the Medical Officer on duty; the hospital was not responsible for providing any special equipment needed; and no special nurses or nursing would be available. At another time it was mentioned that alcoholic drinks were to be paid for by the patients, except for brandy!

In 1926, the Prudential Assurance Co. offered a donation of £20 per annum; it had to be explained that this was not sufficient to endow a bed, the minimum for which was £150; but a small plaque was allowed.

There had been many substantial bequests and donations apart from those already mentioned. By 1908 five beds had been endowed for £1,000 each and six cots similarly and during the war there was a legacy of £3,000 from Miss E.H. Mortimer. Nevertheless, by 1932 it was averred that the hospital's capital reserve was almost exhausted and various emergency measures were recommended:-

1. The almoner (Mr. Wilson) should ensure that there was no exploitation of services in out-patients and should seek voluntary contributions.

2. Prescriptions for insured persons should be provided by chemists rather than from the hospital dispensary.

3. Appeals for annual subscription and more voluntary subscriptions for non-insured patients should be made.

4. The possibility of tax rebate on subscriptions guaranteed for seven years (the modern covenanting).

5. The next year a charge of one shilling was to be made for each X-ray examination.

6. Finally, a new contributory scheme was to be considered.

It was this contributory scheme, which was said to be widely used elsewhere, and which was master-minded by Aubrey Wickham, then the Treasurer who later became Chairman, which proved, it seems, the salvation of the hospital. The scheme was introduced after consultation with representatives, especially from Oxford. It called for regular small contributions from all those in the area served by the hospital who were considered financially able to pay; the rate was 3d a week for a married couple with children under 14; for children aged 14 to 19 an extra penny a week; for a single person tuppence a week. No charge was asked for from old age pensioners or from the 'necessitous poor'; those liable for subscriptions were married couples with more than £5 weekly, or single persons with more than £4 weekly. Benefits from treatment were to be available after subscriptions had been paid for six months - the benefits of course being free inpatient or out-patient treatment. Those who were outside the scheme or had not contributed for six months were expected to pay for their treatment according to their income.

This scheme must have involved a great deal of office work and required much publicity; but it seems to have been an immediate and outstanding success. During the year 26,000 members had joined; 44 local committees had been set up to support the scheme, a number which must surely have covered every town and village on the Island; and a number of employers had undertaken to deduct contributions from their employees (one hopes and assumes with their consent). Cowes alone remained outside the scheme, - presumably because with the Frank James Hospital they felt they could fairly do so. The scheme produced £8,096 in the first year, 1935, and in that year income exceeded expenditure by £3,800. (Besides the sum from the contributory scheme, ordinary income would of course have included some other items such as payment from private patients and for children referred by the Education Department; interest on investments; and donations and bequests). Letters of recommendation after 85 years were discontinued and used no more; anyone receiving treatment who was not already a contributor was expected to become so if they could afford it. Expenses were paid for contributors who had to go into other hospitals; money arising in this way was paid out to the Isle of Wight County Council for patients in Newport Hospital, to the Arthur Webster Hospital and Scio House in Shanklin, to the Royal Southants Hospital and to some London hospitals.

Inevitably the relief was temporary. The next few years and the war, brought a fresh rise in costs, - drugs for example increased in price from £691 in 1936 to £1,660 in 1940. The drug commonly known as M.B. 693 had cost the hospital £60 that year. In 1941 the subscription rate was increase to 5d weekly for man and wife and children up to 14; and old age pensioners were asked to pay a penny a week. At this time under the scheme payment was made to St. Mary's Hospital, Newport at the rate of 6 shillings weekly for abnormal midwifery cases; 15 shillings weekly for acute cases up to ten weeks and 15 shillings weekly for chronic cases up to six weeks; the implication being that chronic cases were properly the business of St. Mary's. During the war the income level at which contributions were expected was raised from £260 to £420 per year. A legacy from Miss Cross in 1942 of £4,238 went towards the extinction of the outstanding debt on the nurses' home.

During the years of the E.M.S., the Ministry had, - sometimes belatedly, - made substantial contributions to the hospital's running expenses. After the war the contributory scheme was continued and many worked hard to promote it and to keep the hospital's finances in hand, but now it was a losing battle; by the middle of 1946 the overdraft was increasing by £1,000 a month. A special appeal for £50,000 was launched, the retired assistant matron, Mrs. Scrimshaw and other nursing staff organising activities among others; out-patients were asked to pay for some of the expensive drugs, - insulin, penicillin and liver extracts. In 1947 the Chairman of the Finance Committee visited the Ministry of Health and it was agreed that the Ministry would contribute £10,000 towards the hospital. This must have been almost on the eve of the N.H.S.

Over the years a great many voluntary efforts were made and it seems fair that these should be recorded. In 1868 and years after amateur theatricals often brought in several pounds. In 1900 Lady Eleanor Cochrane organised and carried through a house to house collection on the Island. More than £700 was collected. In the same year Colonel Gardiner's blind sheep dog 'Blind Jo' collected on the golf links. In 1901 a mother's cot was named after Mrs. Morgan who had collected or given £300. In 1913 Alexandra Day collections, which will be well within the memory of some, were instituted and named after Alexandra, the Queen Mother widow of Kind Edward VII. In 1910 the Matron was given permission to hold a 'Pound Day'. The idea was that gifts of a pound of something or other should be brought to the hospital and the first 'Pound Day' produced 60lb of tea, 12lb of biscuits, 34lb of sugar, 10lb of cocoa, 8lb of coffee, 40lb of soap, 60lb of jam, 6lb of butter and also 22 bottles of port and £6-11-6d in money. It must have been considered a great success. In 1916 the Mayor gave the hospital the takings from the bathing huts at Ryde, £40 odd which he rounded up to £50. In 1928 a bazaar raised £1,450 for the reconstruction fund; in 1929 the Matron introduced 'a birthday fund'; the idea of this was that on an individual's birthday he or she should make a donation to the hospital. In 1931 the hospital was the subject of the B.B.C.'s week's good cause and in the same year Sister Scrimshaw with other sisters and nurses undertook to arrange fund-raising concerts throughout the Island; and in 1933 the H.S.A. undertook to contribute for each of its members six shillings daily if they were an in-patient, and three for an out-patient attendance, and 10-6d for an X-ray. In the same year the Chairman himself collected £507 towards the new X-ray equipment. Before this, round about the turn of the century 'Promenade' concerts had been held at St. Clare, and Calico Balls were held annually; the title of these suggests that they were in marquees, but in fact they were, on occasions anyhow, in the town hall. These contributions and no doubt many others, often small or even trivial in amount, nevertheless collectively added up to a substantial sum, and perhaps more important than that must have helped to engender the mutual regard between the hospital and the population of the Island and of Ryde in particular. It is of course such feelings that lead to the bitter protests when ultimately the time for closure comes.

Figures 1, 2 & 3, Ground Plans, not showing any interior divisions.
These are copies of Ordnance Survey Maps of 1862, 1908 and 1939.
They show progressive stages in the development of the Royal County Hospital.

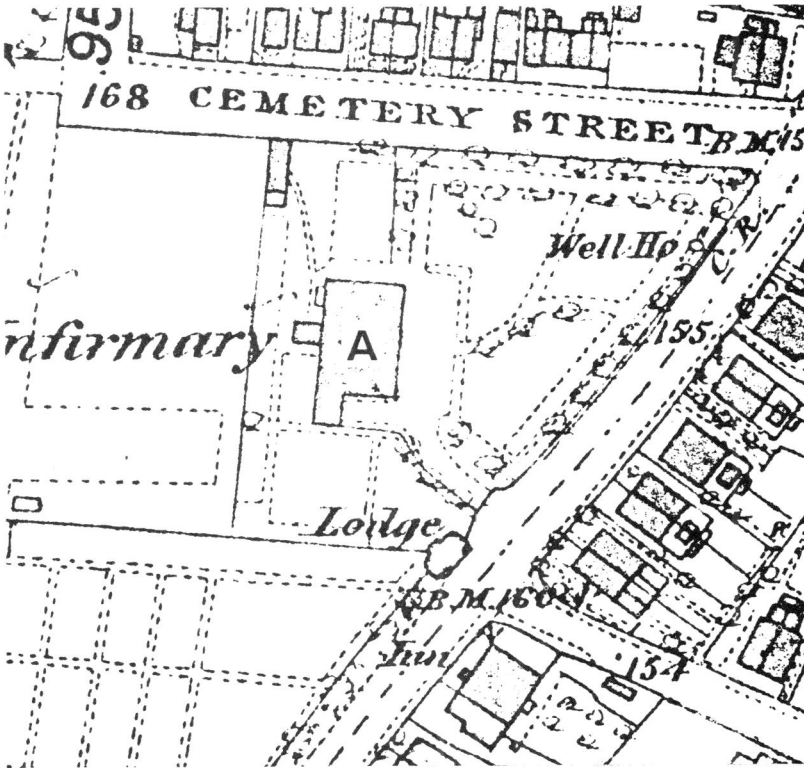

**Figure 1.** Shows the original central block A with small additions at the back (the laundry?) and on the south side (the Out-patients room?). Cemetry Street later became Milligan Street. West Street did not then extend beyond Cemetry Street. *Courtesy: Ordnance Survey.*

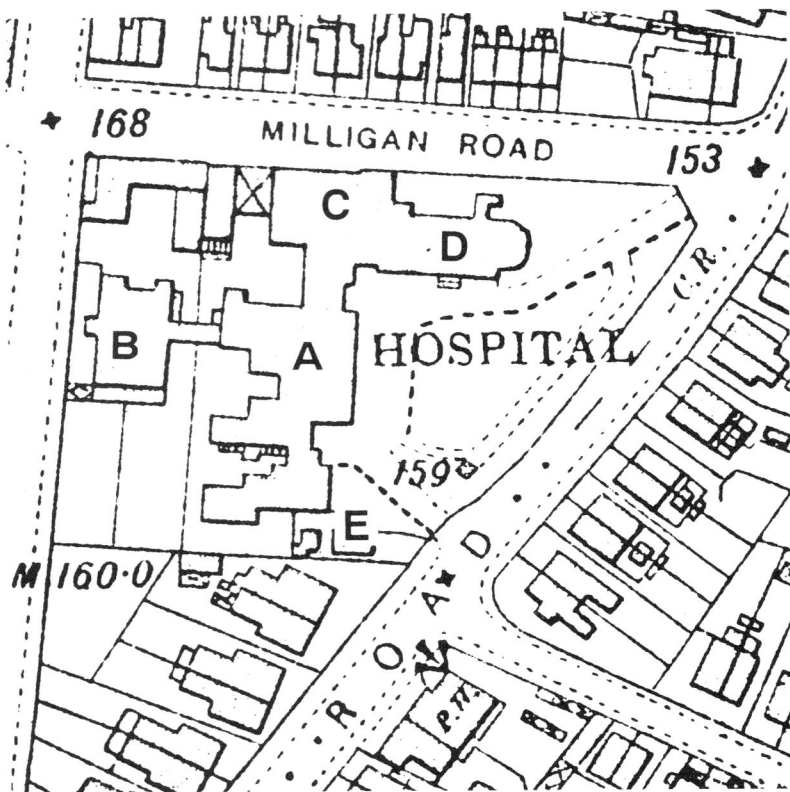

**Figure 2.** There have been many additions.
B is the Milligan (Convalescent) Home.
C the Out-patient and Casualty department.
D is the Queen Victoria Childrens' Ward.
E is the lodge where George Dash lived.
The upper floor of C provided the wards for infectious diseases.
Behind C (i.e. to the west) was the back entrance; mortuary and mortuary chapel;
laundry and boiler house. *Courtesy: Ordnance Survey.*

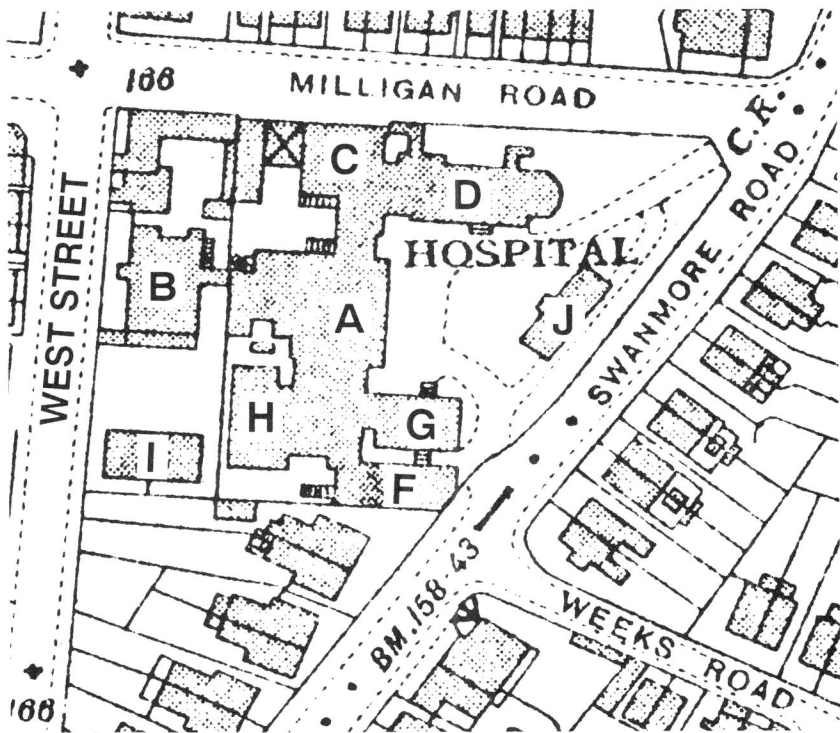

**Figure 3.** Further addtions have been made.
The Lodge has been demolished and replaced by:
F the X-ray department.
G & H are Cottle and Harington wards.
I was, I believe a nurses' home; later with additions and connections it became the Out-patient department with an entrance from West Street.
J is the Pathology laboratory.
The entrance to C is now bricked up with a small window in its upper part. Above this the words 'Out-patient Entrance' can be seen in the masonry.
The West Street entrance to B has above it the memorial tablet to Robert and Elizabeth Milligan. *Courtesy: Ordnance Survey.*

# III

# THE HOUSE OF INDUSTRY (1771)
# THE WORKHOUSE AND INFIRMARY (1864)
# FOREST HOUSE (1904)
# ST. MARY'S HOSPITAL (1935)

To Islanders, St. Mary's has, I believe, seemed a very different type of institution from the Royal I.o.W. County Hospital, - at least until recent years and the N.H.S. Yet they have some things in common; both were founded through the initiative of those who would have been considered, and who considered themselves, the leading citizens of the Island, with a right and duty to decide what was needed; both were intended - in the first place - to serve especially or exclusively the sick and the poor.

It is true of course that they have a very different history. Until its foundation, the care of the aged and destitute, - those unable to support themselves - had, since the time of Elizabeth I, - devolved upon the individual parishes; such people found shelter in the 'Parish House', - accommodation which varied; some parishes had by the time we are thinking of developed a reasonable service and decent living quarters; others less so; some would have been kindly treated, - others perhaps harshly; those who had any capacity for work provided a convenient pool of cheap labour for farmers and others especially at busy times such as harvests.

In 1770, at a meeting of the gentlemen of the Island it was decided that a 'House of Industry' should be erected, - one central building with a salaried staff, where all such people would be accommodated. It was thought that this would provide more effective relief for those who 'by reason of age, infirmities or disease were unable to support themselves, and a better employment of the able and industrious and the education of children'. They thought that by suitable training of the young, these people would become less of a burden to the public.

They placed an advertisement in the *Salisbury Journal* of October 8th 1770, announcing their intention; they obtained 80 acres of Parkhurst Forest from the Crown on a 999 year lease at the nominal rent of £8-17s-9$^{1}/_{2}$d. The House of Industry was modelled on a smaller similar building erected a few years earlier in Sandford in East Suffolk; however in its size and scope, dealing with the

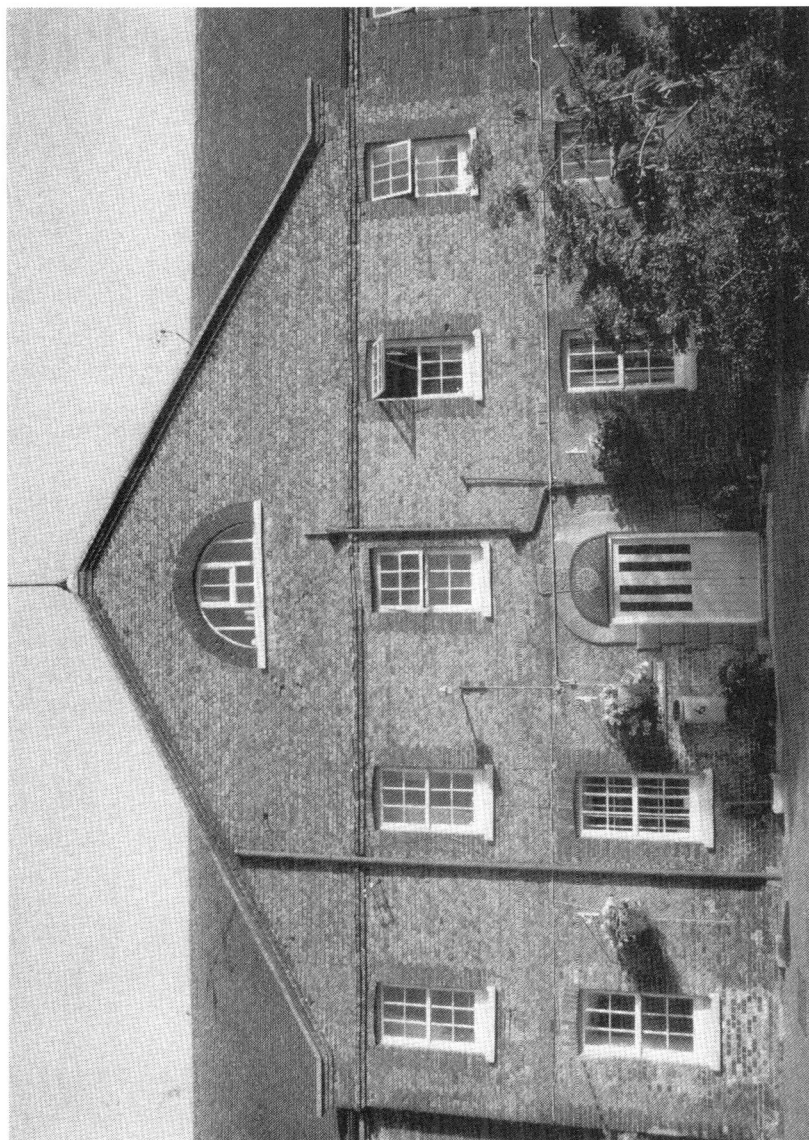

**Plate 7.** House of Industry - now the entrance to St. Catherine's Ward, this must have been at first the main entrance to the House. *Courtesy: Jack Jones.*

whole population of a large area, - the Newport House of Industry was a pioneer development.

As was to be expected, several of the 28 parishes on the Island, - presumably including those which had produced the most advanced services, - opposed the whole idea and there was argument and counter argument, but criticism and opposition were overcome and an Act of Parliament authorised the project in 1771, with a loan of £12,000; a few years later, in the style which is now so familiar, this proved inadequate and a second Act permitted a further £8,000; however by that time the House had been partly built and was occupied - since 1774.

The complex of buildings, - well known to the Island as the House of Industry, the Workhouse, Forest House, more colloquially the Grubber, and finally as St. Mary's, with the upper and lower hospitals, now become the north and south hospitals, - was well described by Worsley in his *History of the Island*, and much of what I write about its early days is derived from his book or from the book by Jack & Johanna Jones *The Isle of Wight; an Illustrated History*; I'm glad to acknowledge the help I have had from both these.

It is said that the familiar pond (now the lake) at St. Mary's was formed in the hollow left when clay was excavated for the bricks which were to be used in the building of the House; I have been unable to find any written evidence of this but it seems likely enough; the pond at first was larger than now, early maps (see figure 4) show it a rectangle about 80 yards x 40 yards; it drained then as now by a stream across Dodnor Lane and through the fields down to the river. The land at the bottom of the hill would have been damp and possibly boggy; there used to be a withy-bed where now car parks slope down to a ditch; but there seems no particular reason why a deep pond should have developed there if it were not man made.

The buildings were near the southern end of the land obtained; Worsley writes:-

'The main building running from east to west, 300ft x 27ft, is of three storeys; about halfway along an extension on the north side 50ft x 21ft provided the chapel, - with a store over it; about 200ft from the west end a wing 170ft x 24ft ran southward at a right-angle to the main building, and from the end of this wing workshops ran westward, parallel to the main building, enclosing a space open on the west side, 200ft x 170ft; to the east of the wing was a courtyard bounded on the north by the main building, on the south by a wall; and on the east by various offices, - dairy, wash-house, brew-house, wood-house, store-rooms, etc.; behind these offices was a barn, a stable and a pig sty.

'In the principal building is a large store room, steward's room, committee room, dining hall 118ft x 27ft, and a common sitting-room for the impotent and aged poor. Under the east end were cellars for beer and meat, 80ft long x 27ft wide; over this building [i.e. on the upper floors] are the laundry, governor's and matron's lodging rooms, nurseries and a sick ward. In the wing on the ground floor are the school room, an apothecary's shop, kitchen and scullery, bakehouse, bread room, governor's and matron's sitting-rooms, pantry, etc. Over are the lying-in rooms, sick wards, and 20 separate rooms or apartments for married men and their wives; with two common sitting-rooms for the old and infirm who lodge in these rooms and are unable to go downstairs.

'In the centre of the workshops before-mentioned..., is a large gateway, on the east side of which is a master weaver's room and a spinning room 96ft x 18ft with store room above; at the west side of the gateway is the shoe-maker's shop, a tailor's shop, and spinning room, 150ft x 18 wide, with weaving room and store rooms over it.

'The House is capable of containing near 700 people; the number supported in it is 500 to 550; it varies with the season and as the county is more or less healthy. Suppose the number to be 550 the proportion will be - of men 64; women 136; girls nine years old and upwards 84; under nine 95; boys nine years old and upwards 56; under that age 116.

'The domestic officers are a governor, matron, steward and school master, who are chosen annually; a chaplain who does duty in the House twice a week besides Sunday. There are also two surgeons and apothecaries and a secretary and treasurer, all of whom except the treasurer had settled salaries.'

The first surgeon (doctor) appointed was Mr. Richard Bassett of Newport who continued until 1795 when he was succeeded by his son who carried on until 1837, being joined for part of this time by Dr Waterworth and Dr Wavell; the first apothecaries were Barlow & Son.

It may be questioned whether, at this early stage the House of Industry could properly be regarded as a hospital; it seems best however to give at least a brief account of it, paying little attention to the Workhouse moiety, interesting though that may be; for from the start it did provide medical and nursing care for the elderly, sick and crippled; from the start too, a medical officer was appointed, and from 1835 onwards he was required to examine everyone admitted to the H.o.I.; in addition sufferers from some infectious diseases were admitted and treated and the institution was for a long time the only place on the Island which offered such care; and thirdly the House very early became a home for those classified as insane, - or as idiots or imbeciles; these terms, and the description of their accommodation as the 'Idiot Wards', sound strange and perhaps offensive to us now as does even the term lunatic asylum; but it should not, I think, be assumed that their care and treatment were lacking in humanity as it was understood at the time. There is plenty of evidence in the records of the concern that was felt for these people and of the endeavours to provide for them reasonable comfort and decent standards.

The House of Industry was managed by 24 Directors and 36 Acting-guardians. Worsley writes:-

'The persons constituting the corporation and styled by the Act Guardians of the Poor are such inhabitants of the Island as are seized in fee, or for life, of their own or their wives rights of land rated to the poor rate of £50 per annum; heirs apparent to £100 per annum; all rectors and vicars; and the occupiers of land rated ... at £100 per annum. Out of the persons thus qualified ... are chosen yearly by ballot 24 Directors, and 36 Acting-guardians who divide and sub-divide themselves into quarterly, monthly and weekly committees of regulation and management ...'

**Figure 4.** (facing page) From the Ordnance Survey of 1862. The House of Industry (here called the Union Workhouse) is at the bottom left hand corner. The fourth (west) side of the quadrilateral shows a continuous building, with projections into the courtyard, which is divided into two parts: the smaller part has trees on two sides.
The building adjacent to the Burial Ground was called the Pest-house in Worsley's day: later it was the Lower Hospital, or, in 1880, the 'Present Infirmary Wards'. The small building further up, marked 'Hospital' and numbered 115 must at this stage have been the Infectious Diseases Hospital.
135 & 135a are ponds which drain across Dodnor Lane and down to the river, as now.
The small rectangular building between the north and west wings of the H of I was what in those days was called 'the Necessaries'.
The small buildings near Dodnor Lane were farm buildings. *Courtesy: Ordnance Survey.*

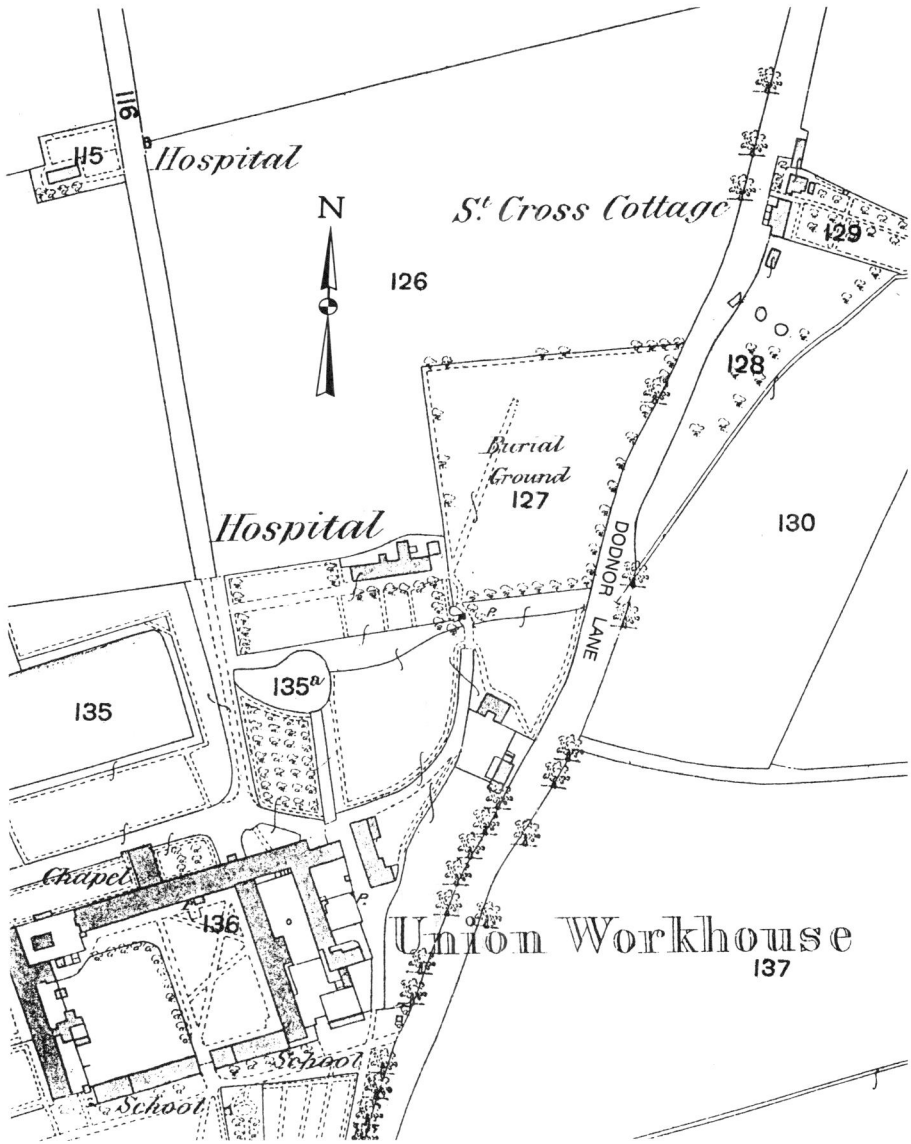

Figure 4

The Directors were in fact the managers, and they were drawn from the land owners and the Clergy, the original initiators of the Act; the Acting-guardians were answerable to them, and were selected as representatives of the parishes; the House, built by a loan, was dependent on the parish rates for its day to day running. Both Directors and Guardians took their duties seriously; they could be, and on occasions were, fined for failing to attend the committee meetings.

J. & J. Jones write that the Directors became the driving force of local Government on the Island; besides managing the House, they dealt with outdoor relief, the collection of rates and in time they supervised some primitive medical service. In 1836, the introduction of the new Poor Law, abolishing the old Elizabethan statutes, meant that they became answerable to the Poor Law Board and Commissioners; - but the management of the House did not greatly change; in 1865 the Poor Law Board dissolved the 'incorporation', and the Isle of Wight Union was established, first meeting on September 28th 1865, and a Board of Guardians now managed the House of Industry although its personnel was very much the same as had been the previous management; and in 1871 the Poor Law Board itself gave way to the Local Government Board; all the activities of the Guardians had to be confirmed by this Board - e.g. even the appointment of a nurse or a domestic worker; and all new buildings or alterations must be approved by it. The Local Government Board itself gave way to the Ministry of Health in 1919, and the Guardians were finally dissolved and their function taken over by the County Council in 1930; the Council then already managed Whitecroft and Longford Hospitals on the Island; then after another two decades came the N.H.S.

The House of Industry had this in common also with the Ryde Hospital, - that in both of them building, additions and alterations to the initial structure, seemed almost continuous. Very few plans are now available; a few of alterations in the House and a few showing the design of the new wards in 1880-1882 which came to form what was later known to us as the upper hospital; those apart, the only available information is in the maps of the ordnance surveys, from which a ground plan of the buildings can be obtained; the first survey in 1810 was not of the same standard as later maps; but the surveys about 1860 and 1940 give useful evidence of the existing buildings and they are shown in figures 4 and 5. I shall try to describe the development of the various buildings as time went on and hope that the figures will go some way to showing how they ended up as the hospital we have known.

The first new building was an isolated unit for smallpox put up in 1782, and it seems there was additional provision for this in 1794. In those years smallpox was evidently the infection which most urgently called for isolation. Other infections at first were treated in the 'Pest-house' as its name implied; Scarlet Fever, Typhoid Fever, and Cholera are mentioned.

The 'Pest-house' was built at the same time as the House of Industry and is mentioned by Worsley in his book published in 1781; he says it was situated about three to four hundred yards from the main building; it lay to the east of the path or drive which then, and still now, leads up the hill to the buildings further up; it must have been approximately where there is now a temporary car park and just below the recently levelled helicopter pad; it became known as the Lower Hospital, as will be told, and it was not demolished until about 1952, although it had been for a long time then out of use. (It was not until 1948 that the Workhouse itself (Forest House) was referred to as the 'Lower Hospital'; by that time the Pest-house had long been out of use for patients: part of it, I am told, was a carpenter's shop). Adjacent was the burial ground; this was enlarged later, the Bishop of Portsmouth consecrating it at that time, and there is a note in 1854 about the path leading from the chapel to the 'Pest-house' where the mortuary was built, and the burial ground; in 1867 graves in the burial ground were all to be marked and numbered and a record kept in a book.

The need for care of the insane also arose very early; in 1784 two places of confinement, - or cells, - were provided and four more not later than 1810; by 1813 a large separate building had been put up, - it was this building which, more or less, filled in the fourth side of the quadrilateral of buildings that made up the House; it was enlarged in 1822 and again in 1830; by 1832 there were 28 inmates; the Guardians had earlier in 1832 had to obtain a licence authorising them to retain lunatics in the House.

In the 'Pest-house' separate wards had been set aside for Venereal Disease, and also for the Itch; but in 1834 all this department dealing with infectious diseases was moved to the building which had been set up near the top of the hill, reached by a path or drive which must have been the same as the path which now leads up to the stores and the former kitchen, restaurant and Pathology Department. This seems to have been a very small building, and one cannot visualise it holding more than about half a dozen beds, - or if it was of two storeys perhaps eight or ten. From this time the 'Pest-house' was referred to as the 'Lower Hospital' and it became perhaps the first place on the Island to offer some sort of hospital care for what may be called general medicine and surgery. A list of diagnoses given in 1837 includes injuries, burns, arthritis, and dropsy; of course this hospital was presumably available only for people transferred from the House of Industry. In 1834 a separate ward with a separate entrance was set aside for the treatment of the Itch.

Dr Bassett retired in 1837; he and his father had served the Guardians for some 70 years since the foundation of the House; he himself for about 50 years. Dr Waterworth carried on and in 1840 he reported that the asylum was too small -

'Patients cannot be kept apart, but all must be together; quiet or convalescent patients are disturbed by noisy ones; courtyards are too small and cannot be observed adequately; rooms are dark and damp. Most patients however are clean and happy, and restraint is used as little as possible.'

**Figure 5.** (facing page) This is from the Ordnance Survey map of 1940. Most of the buildings remain now. In the Lower Hospital (H of I) the continuous building across the west side has been replaced by three separate buildings, - which by 1994 became Holly House, the Diabetic Centre and the Secretaries House.

The building opposite Forest Road, with the former entrance to the hospital grounds, was demolished when the relief road and roundabout were built. The 'new' entrance a little way up the road towards Cowes has the Porter's Lodge, with weigh-bridge, just inside it, and the reception wards (which became offices) running eastward along the drive.

The old Pest-house is still there, roughly where now is a car-park; it was not at this stage in use as hospital accommodation, - not I think since about 1880.

The Upper Hospital, (or Infirmary) has blocks A & B as later, with the central block providing kitchens, dining rooms and nurses' rooms.

The buildings to the east of Block A separated by a path were the lying-in (obstetric) wards: north of that the old infectious disease wards: with modifications and additions the former of these would become Carisbrooke Ward and the dental surgery - and later the surgical day hospital: and the latter, the theatre and surgical ward (Bonchurch): the corridor joining these two to the main hospital was built about 1942. The mortuary with its chapel-of-ease north of these two, replaced the smaller, older I.D. Hospital, which had been demolished.

Hassall ward came to lie to the west of the hospital: the Obstetric wing to the north-west, and the new kitchens and dining-room, pathology laboratory, stores, and finally Newcroft, north and north-east - between them dwarfing the earlier buildings. *Courtesy: Ordnance Survey.*

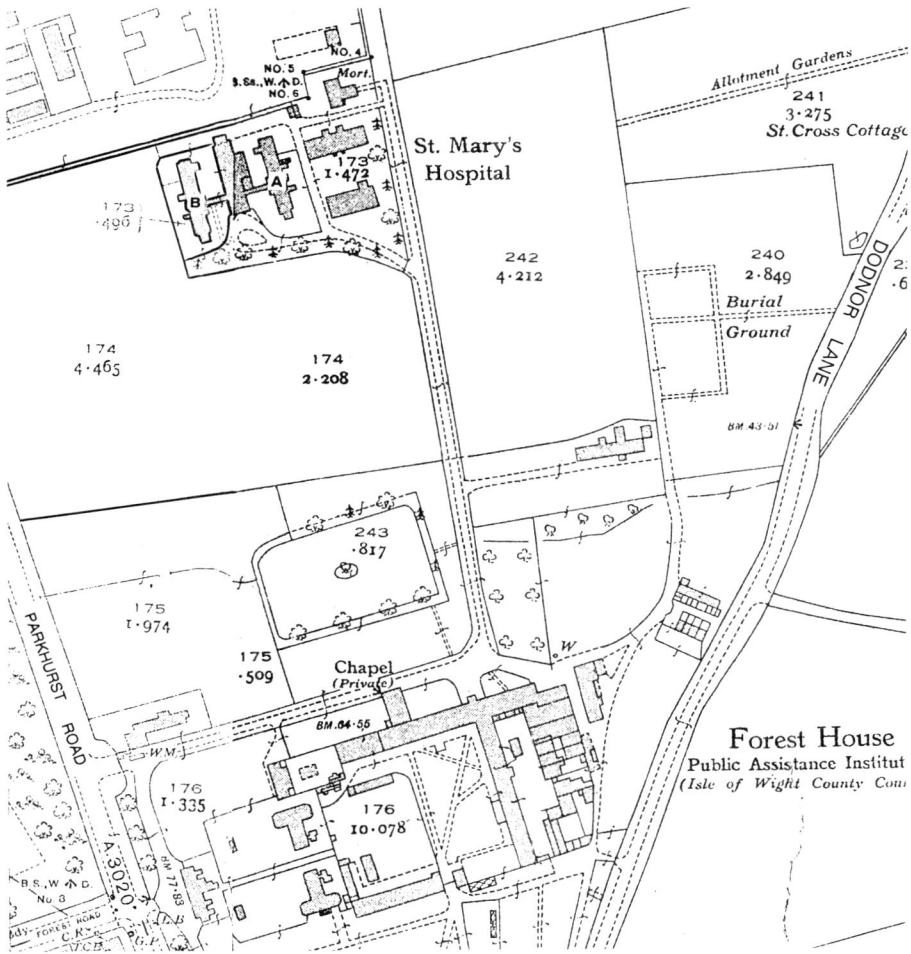

**Figure 5**

At that time there were 12 men and 22 women in residence. Much earlier about 1810 a small number of women had been sent to an asylum in Laverstock where they were under the care of a Dr Finch, and now a few more were sent there, but some years later the Guardians, when asked, denied any need for any comprehensive transfer of patients to the Hampshire County Asylum at Knowle.

In that same year the doctors collectively asked that, in the interest of both the profession and the public, all doctors might be admitted at any time to the hospital to see and study hospital practice; likewise all apprentices, pupils and assistants; and that notice should be given of all operations to be performed in order that they might attend and observe. This request was refused by the Guardians, - possibly one of their less enlightened decisions; but they did accept a motion calling upon the surgeon to the House to show every consideration to other medical officers. Bureaucracy was in the ascendant about this time; doctors were required to indicate on their returns a visit, a call, or a supply of medicine to a patient, by the letters V, C, or M; the surgeon to the House was required to make a daily record of all sick in the House, using the form of the Poor Law Union, which was to be produced at the weekly committee meetings; and doctors were instructed in 1849 that no new patient should receive medicine more than once, unless the M.O. had visited to determine the effect of the medicine. In 1828 it had been ordered that the three surgeons attending the hospital (Bassett, Wavell, and Waterworth) should all be present and consulted before any operation took place. Wiser perhaps and more indicative of genuine care was the rule in 1837 that no patient was to be transferred from the hospital to the House in a dying state (suggesting that even then there was pressure on beds and concern about turnover) and some years later, that any patient requiring attention during the night should be transferred to the hospital.

The Governor complained in 1842 that the hospital accommodation was inadequate and during this decade it was improved. Bathrooms and a new water tank were built for the Upper Hospital and a new mortuary was added to the Lower. More building went on and more equipment was acquired for the hospital, including three thermometers, a water bed and two water cushions; twelve ear trumpets; knives and forks and trenchers for the asylum; and later counterpanes and a mercurial vapour lamp. Over the years also the Guardians received several boxes of linen from Col. Biddulph at Osborne by order of the Queen; games and toys were received for the children; and bibles and prayer books were purchased in 1850 and the Rev. McAlb provided communion plate.

Albany Barracks, on the west side of the Cowes road, had been built about half a century earlier in the time of the Napoleonic Wars; the drainage tended naturally to pass through the hospital grounds on its way down to the river, and there was a number of exchanges between the military and the Guardians with claims and counter claims; in 1848 there was concern about drainage of the cesspool at the barracks and the Guardians declined to pay part of the cost of this drainage. In 1861 there was a complaint that alterations made would divert part of the drainage into the hospital pond; later Major Robinson produced a plan for the drainage through an open ditch running through the Workhouse garden but avoiding the pond, which was accepted.

An epidemic of Cholera occurred on the Island (and elsewhere) in 1849; it was then that the Guardians thanked the committee of the Royal Isle of Wight Infirmary for the offer of two wards for a cholera hospital; such an offer, made while the hospital was still being built, must one feels have indicated a real emergency; the Guardians undertook, if agreeable, to provide furniture for the wards. I can find no evidence however in the records about the hospital that the offer of accommodation was actually taken up although one cannot be sure that it was not so; the Guardians also thanked the Ryde doctors and chemists for their help and they made an award to Driver Smeddle and his assistant Welch who, when others refused, offered to convey a patient from Ryde to Newport; they gave gratuities to the staff, medical and nursing, who attended the patients, and a grant of £50 to Arthur Clarke, - Clerk to the Guardians for the work he had done during the epidemic.

The licence authorising the 'Carisbrooke Asylum' to retain patients there expired in 1853, and the Guardians were asked where the patients should go; the question must have been anticipated for a few patients had already been transferred to the House of Industry and the previous year Dr Ferguson of the Hampshire County Asylum had asked for the names of patients; now in spite of previous rejection of the need they arranged for the transfer of 20 women and several men to Knowle in Hampshire. The Isle of Wight Steam Packet offered a special steamer for the move, at a charge of seven guineas, - an offer which was accepted. This was not of course the end of the asylum. Several patients were retained and some, regarded as harmless and incurable, returned from Knowle; but it gave an opportunity for another re-planning and rebuilding of the asylum wards, and a sub committee produced a plan to provide a male and female receiving ward, an 'Idiot Ward', and a residence for the chaplain; mentioning that as far as possible, the building work should be done by the inmates of the House of Industry.

It was nevertheless, about this time that the matron complained that the number of women resident in the House was becoming so reduced that she had difficulty in getting the laundry done. Improved equipment for the laundry was provided; and a few years later the Master likewise needed more help with farming because of the small number of men available and purchase of a plough was allowed. It seems that the House of Industry with its sick wards and cripple wards and with the increasing demand on the asylum and the hospital, was becoming more a hospital and rather less of a workhouse; moreover the boys' accommodation over the school room was abolished and the boys moved elsewhere.

The House had its first royal visit in 1869; Queen Victoria accompanied by the Dowager Duchess of Atholl and Lt.-General Seymour visited the Union Workhouse and was pleased to express the strongest approbation of the good order and cleanliness which pervaded every department. It was I think after this that she presented the House with a quilt, - of which more is told later.

Worries on the part of the medical officers about ventilation, drainage, and the adequacy of accommodation continued. In 1871-72 an epidemic of smallpox occurred on the Island and Dr Beckingsale received a bonus of £15 for his work during this. In 1872 the Guardians decided (with some opposition) to put up a new building with 24 hospital beds; the Local Government Board which had now replaced the Poor Law Board was critical of the plans, and demanded many changes which the Guardians complained were at variance with the advice and information they had from their medical officers; they asked for an inspector to come and confer; but they had instead to send a deputation to London; new plans were made and agreed; money was to be raised by an increase in parish rates; debate continued through much of 1873, but in September, the new building was postponed indefinitely and W.T. Stratton, a Newport Architect, produced plans for the improvement of the Lower Hospital which were accepted.

This was however only a temporary postponement; by the end of the decade in 1879, a new building was again on the agenda; the Local Government Board was glad to hear of this, and accepted the Guardians' assertion that the present lying-in wards, which had been improved, but remained for another 25 years in the House of Industry, were adequate.

Dr E. Waterworth, by now the medical officer in succession to Dr Beckingsale, was asked to comment on the number of beds needed; in his report on the House of Industry and the Lower Hospital he showed that there were in the hospital 3 wards for men with 5, 5 and 9 beds and also 1 for Venereal Disease with 5 beds; for the women 2 wards with 4 and 10 beds and 1 for Venereal Disease with 6 beds; in the House, nurses and 'wardsmen' slept in the sick wards with the residents. They were themselves of course residents promoted to this work; the mens' garret provided 18 beds plus 2 for wardsmen; the 'inner sick room' 22 plus 2; and the 'outer sick room' was a passage room with 12 beds but no provision for a nurse; the womens' sick wards held 15 plus 2 and a cripple ward 14 plus 1; the lying-in ward provided 7 beds with 1 nurse; Dr Waterworth mentioned that cases with 'Fever' and Smallpox were provided for in the Upper Hospital; cases of Itch were at present said to be very rare and were treated in the receiving wards; his recommendation for the new buildings was for 20 mens' beds and 30 womens' beds; also 2 wards with 4 beds for children, and 2 for those with Venereal Disease; and a surgery for operations and examinations and a dispensary.

For the new wards William Tucker Stratton produced three plans; the first was sited on the east side of the drive, four wards in a square with a central court, which would have been built roughly where now the lower part of the stores and the building known until lately as 'Nurses' Home Two' stand; this must have been rejected in favour of a building on the west side of the drive, a bit further to the west and a bit lower down than the existing wards for infectious diseases. This site was approved by the representative of the Local Government Board, Dr Mowat, who came down to confer with the Guardians and the medical officers; it had five buildings joined by a long corridor running east and west; the buildings projecting on either side; the central one a single storey, with offices and administrative quarters on the south side and kitchen and dining room on the north of the corridor. A few yards along the corridor from this central building on either side were single storey buildings with childrens' wards, one for boys and one for girls on the south side and wards for Venereal Disease on the north side, and further along again two-storey buildings with wards upstairs and down, again for men at one end and women at the other. This rather ambitious building was abandoned in favour of a smaller one which merely had a central two storey block with administrative accommodation, kitchens and dining room, joined by corridors to the ward blocks on either side, - the west side for men and the east side for women; this building was slightly further up the hill than the earlier one; the two plans were rather curiously shown together on a single plan (Fig 6); this final plan which was adopted provided upper St. Mary's, as it came to be known, with blocks A and B. The existing wards for infectious diseases - known until then as the Upper Hospital - were alongside this building as shown in the Ordnance Survey Map of 1910.

£7,000 was spent on building these new wards, - a loan from Mr. S.R. Valentine-Robinson of Gresham Street at $4\frac{1}{8}\%$; building proceeded through

1881 though in September a committee felt that progress was slow and urged the contractor to greater expedition; in February 1882 gas lighting for the wards was agreed, and later that year a contract for a steam boiler was settled and £30 was allotted for trees and shrubs around the wards; finally it is clear from the minutes that an 'operating room' was associated with these wards. In January 1883 the Master was given instructions for the wards to be occupied; and a small fire engine was purchased.

These new wards, hereafter known as the Infirmary, presented to the south a facade somewhat resembling the letter E on its side, - with a central entrance and a wing, the paired wards, on either side, - to me slightly reminiscent of the style supposed to be characteristic of that of some of the Island Manor houses; (e.g. Arreton, Merston, Yaverland); one must not press the resemblance too far; these buildings partly enclosed a three sided courtyard with a central tree and a line of evergreen oaks forming a fourth side, where later other buildings were to come.

When opened things did not at first go perfectly smoothly, - a familiar situation with a new untried department, which tends to present unanticipated problems. The windows were unsatisfactory; the chimneys smoked (all heating of the wards at this stage of course was either by open fires or by coke stoves); the hot water system was defective and the supply insufficient; and the nursing accommodation was inadequate. With time and patience no doubt all these matters were dealt with.

**Figure 6.** (facing page) This is the plan for what became the Infirmary, later Upper St. Mary's; now part of the North Hospital. The shaded plan is super-imposed upon an earlier and larger plan which was abandoned. It is approximately, but not precisely, that which was eventually built. The building to the east (right) of the new one, marked 'Present Wards for Infectious Diseases' was earlier referred to as the Upper Hospital. It is not seen in the O.S. map of 1862, which does show the smaller building north of it: this smaller building must for several decades have provided such accommodation as there was for infectious diseases: the larger one not present in 1862 must have been built between then and 1880, the date of this plan. *Courtesy: I.W. County Records Office.*

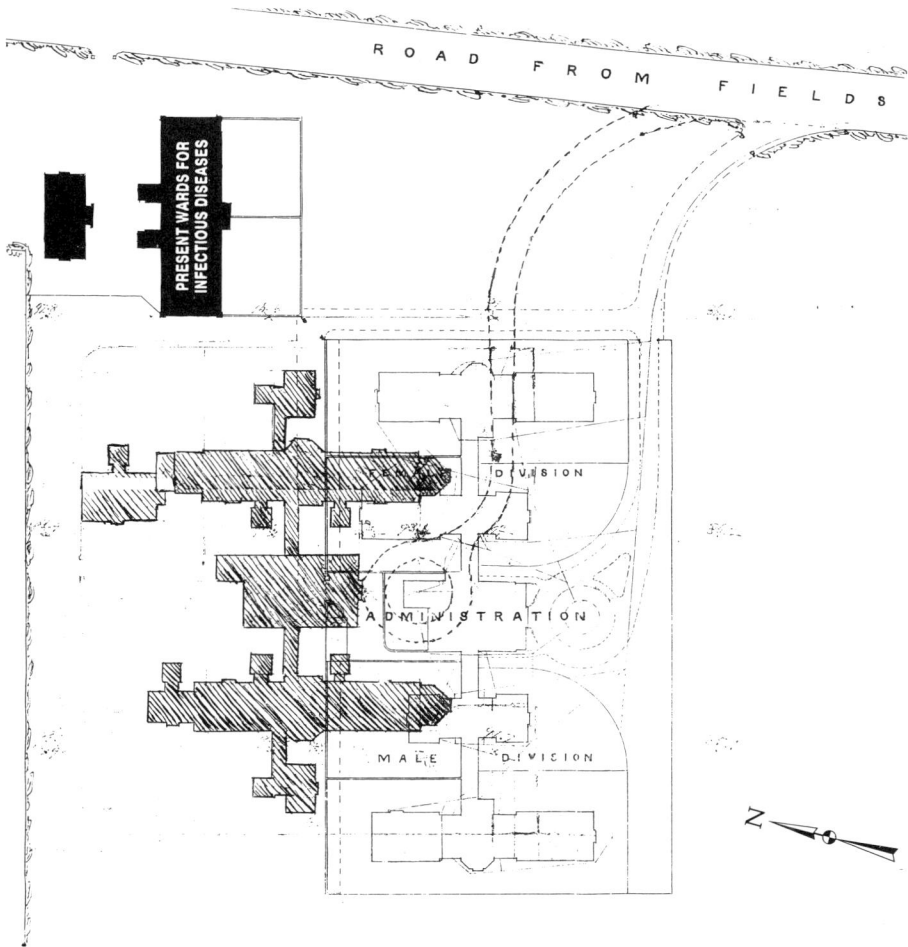

ROAD FROM FIELDS

PRESENT WARDS FOR INFECTIOUS DISEASES

DIVISION

ADMINISTRATION

MALE DIVISION

N

**Figure 6**

Dr Beckingsale, as mentioned, joined the staff in 1846; his retirement in 1877 was a sad episode involving the staff and particularly the nursing and medical staff. A resident of the House had died, and was found by a coroner's jury to have died from starvation, but they were not prepared to say whether this was due to neglect or otherwise; the Guardians asked for a report from the Local Government Board and this was provided by Dr Mowat and Mr. Baldwyn Fleming; their enquiry, on which the report was based, was attended by the Chairman, Vice Chairman, and other committee members. It must have been highly critical, and it demanded the resignation of the medical officer to the House; the Governor was censured, and two nurses dismissed. Dr Beckingsale submitted his resignation which was accepted with great regret; he had served the House for 30 years, during which he had 'Invariably fulfilled his duty in an efficient and skilful manner such to have elicited the unqualified approbation of the Guardians', and they expressed their sympathy with him in the circumstances which led to his resignation. He applied for a superannuation allowance, - but this was disallowed and he withdrew his application; but several months later in 1878 a memorial was submitted signed by 84 property owners and rate-payers, saying they would be glad if the Guardians could in any way manifest their recognition of the doctor's long and faithful service. This was considered by a special committee but did not lead to anything, and in May 1878 a renewed appeal was rejected.

It seems that the infectious disease wards were, in fact, taken over by agreement by the Royal Sanitary Authority, in 1887 - indeed the record implies that there was statutory authority for this; not long after this the R.S.A. asked for, and was granted, permission to store a hospital tent in the House of Industry; one supposes that this was, at the time, the way of solving the difficulty of shortage of beds in an epidemic.

Now in 1889-1890 came the County Council, and the separation of the Isle of Wight from Hampshire. Soon after it came into being the Council offered the Guardians £3,000 for 38 acres of land (which at that time still belonged to the Guardians although much of it would have been leased out for farming), on which they planned to build a mental hospital; this offer was declined.

More new buildings came in 1895, when a plan was adopted to build a new receiving ward, with new entrance to the hospital grounds, immediately opposite the road now known as the Forest Road; at the same time the whole of the imbecile wards were to be re-planned yet again, - the plans being approved by the Local Government Board; this when completed, provided one large building facing the road; with two others back from that forming the fourth side of the quadrilateral, and a third one in line with those two which became the chaplain's house. These buildings, constructed by Mr. Hayles, required a loan of £5,500 in 1897 and an additional one of £1,100 from the ecclesiastical commissioners. To anticipate, the new building close to the road became for a time and at least in part, a residence for the farm bailiff, and later, in the days of the N.H.S. a physiotherapy centre, and then the school for spastic and handicapped children, - Forest-Side School; when the relief road from Newport was built, a large slice of land, now mainly occupied by the roundabout, was taken off the hospital grounds, - chiefly the large flat field known as the cricket ground, and sometimes used for that purpose; and the Forest-Side School was demolished (before this, the Cowes/Newport road ran straight through to Hunnyhill with Forest Road and Whitesmith Road turning off it).

Bells were fitted in the wards in 1895, and better accommodation for night nurses had to be found. Various small matters, - not necessarily unimportant - deserve a mention. The Royal Mail was delivered to the Infirmary separately from the House of Industry. It required some pressure on the Post Office before this was agreed. The Chairman and Vice Chairman attended a conference of hospital administrators seeking a reduction in telephone charges (one can guess the result). The Guardians agreed to the erection of telephone poles on their ground, - charging one shilling per annum per pole. A dentist was appointed to the staff in 1900. In 1891 the committee had made a charge of tuppence per person for skating on the hospital pond (there is, may-be, a hint here for a hard pressed Finance Officer). Later there was correspondence with the fishing club in Newport about fishing rights on the pond. In 1910 an extension of the central (administrative) building of the Infirmary gave improved accommodation, on two floors, for nurses.

A committee of ladies was appointed in 1895 though probably for the House of Industry rather than the Infirmary; a suggestion 'That great good might result from the attendance of a committee of ladies (under the control of the chaplain)' had been made so far ago as 1835, but it was not for 60 years that this one was actually appointed. A majority of Guardians, after debate, voted that the medical officers' prescriptions should be examined by the Guardians!

The water supply had, from the start of the House of Industry been a problem, and it continued so, - there was a well in the courtyard with a pump house (the building is still there) and there is frequent comment in the minutes about the building and deepening of the well, the functioning of the pump, and the purity of the water. In December 1904, the Works Committee reported that after many difficulties, and expenditure of £494, the well was now in perfect order and should fulfil the needs for the years to come.

In 1902 Princess Beatrice, Governor of the Island, paid a formal visit. She toured the House, with a pause for presentation and speeches in the Board Room; she then took afternoon tea in the master's drawing room, when the Matron was presented; then on to the Infirmary, both mens' and womens' wards, which were found to be 'Delightfully light and airy'; the oldest lady patient had on her bed the quilt presented years earlier by Queen Victoria. Later this quilt was framed and hung in the Board Room, behind the Chairman's seat, and in 1905 a brass plate was fixed below it given anonymously through Mr. Dabell; eventually it found its way to the Carisbrooke Museum. No separate mention is made of the lying-in wards which were still then in the House, but in 1904 they were transferred to the Infirmary. Shortly before this the Guardians had decreed that the House should be renamed Forest House, and this name appears on the Ordnance Survey Map of 1910; this meant that children born there would not hence-forth have to be recorded as having been born in the Workhouse.


Regular inspections were made by the Local Government Board, - the Inspector for several years being Mr. Baldwyn Fleming already mentioned. His reports were generally favourable, and indeed became almost effusive in 1905, - 'During my inspection I found the Workhouse generally in very good order; I observed many and most useful alterations and improvements. The condition of the Infirmary is especially satisfactory. No complaint was made to me. I shall have great pleasure in informing the Local Government Board of the care and kindly feeling with which the Guardians and their officers supply the needs of the poor.' Despite this good report, - repeated by Mr. Baldwyn Fleming until 1909, - when he retired, the Coroner holding an inquest in that year on a patient who died after an accident, expressed the opinion that the hospital was considerably under-staffed, in view of the fact that one nurse had been in charge of 13 wards, male and female, at the time of the accident. (It is in parenthesis difficult to see how this figure of 13 could have been made up; eight wards, would seem to be a maximum; perhaps some were divided). The Guardians in due course conferred with the Local Government Board, and decided to increase the nursing officers from seven to eight!

Smallpox was always a problem for the hospitals, Ryde as well as Newport, and later for the isolation or fever hospitals. After the Infirmary was separated from these infectious disease wards, it did not often crop up again, but in 1890 one case was admitted because of the impossibility of finding room anywhere else. Vaccination against Smallpox was a different matter; in country areas especially it may be that there was reluctance to accept it even when it became legally compulsory; on the Island the resistance seems to have been extreme; again and again Medical Officers, and Relieving Officers, reported the near impossibility of persuading people to accept it. In 1856 it was suggested that the Poor Law Board should be informed that the 'Vaccination (compulsory) Act is to a considerable extent inoperative on the Island.' Whether voluntary acceptance improved after the epidemic of 1872 I do not know, but certainly there was still much resistance.

The County Council, in its early years anyhow, favoured the idea of sending cases of Smallpox to a hospital ship in Cowes; whether this actually ever came about I have not been able to determine; but there certainly was a hospital ship, the principal object of which was, one supposes, to look after cases of infectious disease arriving at the port of Cowes. The ship was mentioned recently in the *County Press*, in the column designated '100 Years Ago'. It was referred to there as the 'Cholera Hospital Ship', and at the time (March 1894) was considered to be in a parlous state; but certainly later annual reports of the Medical Officer to the Cowes Port Authority, mentioned it and made recommendations for keeping it in good order.

I have as yet made little mention of nurses and nursing, - it seems to make a more coherent story if it is considered in one section from the start. Jane Adams, one of the earliest matrons, who was in office from 1779 to 1794, was in the view of J. & J. Jones a very able manager, who no doubt established a high standard. Her salary was £30 per annum, and she would have been answerable to the Master (Governor). Nurses in those days of course had no formal training, and required no particular qualifications; they must have been chosen from among the available resident population in the House and any training they did there must have been, quite literally, 'in-house'; and there were not many of them. They did not have any expectation of regular pay; if they had not been nursing they would have had to do some other work anyhow.

The first mention of any appointment of a professional or at least a paid nurse, was the appointment in 1826 of an 'assistant nurse' to superintend the 'hospital', at a salary not exceeding £10 yearly; whether the term 'hospital' at this time referred to the small block near the top of the hill; the larger 'Pest-house', which later became the 'Lower Hospital' or the hospital for the insane and imbeciles, is not clear. There must by then have been some sort of nursing service, since the following year, in January 1827, a gratuity of £5 was to be distributed among the nurses of the hospital (we must again remember that this was something like £250 now in terms of purchasing power). In 1829 the nurses were to have a gratuity of two shillings 'for this quarter only'.

The superintendent of the asylum in 1830 was to receive a salary of £42 a year; and in 1847 there was a recommendation that the matron of the asylum should have £20 a year and should also have the assistance of two male keepers. Later that year nurses in the hospital and the receiving wards were to have 'diet number two', (which I think was the diet given to the working members of the male staff,) except they would be allowed seven pints of beer weekly instead of the fourteen pints supplied to the men; soon after this it was accepted that nurses in the asylum were to have clothing distinct from that of the patients. Ten years later the nurses in the receiving wards were to receive £6 yearly. These nurses must, I think, still have been recruited from among the residents of the House, and this must have been their living place, unless they had rooms off the wards. It is a long time before there is any mention of separate accommodation for nurses, - not in fact until the Infirmary was built. However it is the case that the infectious disease wards did have accommodation for a nurse as did the lying-in wards.

A Cholera epidemic occurred in 1866, and at that time, the nurses as well as the matron, medical officer, Governor and clerk, had an addition to their salaries. The next year in 1867 the appointment of a head nurse at £18 yearly, two male and two female nurses may have been for the infectious disease (or Upper) Hospital, since at the same time advertisements for two nurses in the Lower Hospital at £12 yearly were made, and for a nurse in the idiot ward at £15; whether the higher salary indicates a superior degree of training, experience or presumptive ability, or merely a recognition of the quality of the work, one cannot say. By now however there must surely have been some accommodation set aside for these paid nurses, but where is not clear. Nursing by now however must have been in process of becoming a career and a calling. It was more than a decade after the Crimean War and the work of Florence Nightingale; there is mention that vacancies for nurses sometimes required repeated advertising, and some appointments were made provisional for a month's trial. All appointments had of course to be referred to the Local Government Board, which must have involved a significant delay; in 1873 the Medical Officers were asked to rearrange nursing duties, so that nurses would not be called upon to do domestic work which could be tackled by the servants! In this year paid nurses, (distinct from the inmates of the House of Industry drafted for nursing duties) were to wear uniform dresses.

Two years later in 1875, the Medical Officers recommended and asked for an increase in nursing staff of one male nurse for the idiot wards; one for the inner and outer men's sick wards (in the House); one female nurse for the female cripple ward, and a married couple for the infectious disease hospital; only the first of these five was agreed by the Guardians.

However by 1895, control of Infirmary and the sick wards in the House was to be in the hands of a head nurse or superintendent, independent of the Master, and five years later an assistant matron was appointed, with a salary of £30 (matron's salary at this stage was £45 raised to £60 in 1900). A few years later night attendants for the imbecile wards were arranged.

A letter was received from the Winchester Union with copies of a lecture on 'nursing in the Workhouse' by Mr. Baldwyn-Fleming; copies of this letter were sent to all absent members of the Board. It would be interesting to see this letter, one wonders if any copies are extant. Nursing associations had come into being on the Island, - an association in Ryde was mentioned earlier; and in 1895 the Guardians agreed terms for supplying nurses for the wards. These nursing associations, one supposes, filled the role now filled by nursing agencies.

The lying-in wards were moved from the House of Industry in 1904 to the Infirmary above, and the following year assistant nurses at the Infirmary were to receive training in midwifery. Much earlier in 1875, Dr Castle had offered to instruct a class of women in midwifery, if he could have the necessary equipment; the Local Government Board however at that time barred any additional expenditure on such a service.

'Probationer nurses' were appointed to the Infirmary in 1907 (on the female side); they were to have a salary of £12 yearly rising by £2 a year to £16. The significance of this presumably is that some sort of nurse training was now envisaged; also that accommodation for them must have been available. In June 1910 the Classification Sub Committee of the Guardians (this was the sub committee concerned with personnel, etc.) recommended, for the Infirmary, one superintendent nurse (at £40 to £55 a year ), three trained staff nurses at £30, five probationers (at £12 - £17 - £22), and one male sick attendant at £30. Accommodation was to be provided by extending the first floor of the administration block over the kitchen and surgery. Isle of Wight nurses were to be given preference.

There is little more to be learned from the minutes of the Committee up to 1930 when the County Council took over the House and the Infirmary. During the 1920s there were usually about 80 patients in the Infirmary, - this included the Obstetric Department, and perhaps about 200 in the House and the asylum. In 1913 there was seemingly some adverse criticism of the management of the

Infirmary, and the following year a new appointment of a superintendent nurse was made, but there is no mention of the number of nursing staff.

The term 'surgery', used above in mentioning the extension over the administrative block, is of interest since the 'surgery' was probably the room provided for examinations and operations, and this suggests that the first 'operating room' was in this central block.

The provision of an ambulance was apparently in the first place in the hands of hospitals (and Guardians) rather than of the County Council. A horse-drawn cart had been made available early on, and in 1922 the Guardians accepted gratefully the offer of a horse-drawn ambulance from the Joint Hospital Board; three years after this in 1925 they purchased a motor ambulance from F. Cheverton for £205-1s-6d.

I have not attempted to deal with the history and development of the House of Industry which is outside the scope of this book, apart from its association with the hospital and medical services; but since it was to become the Lower (or now the South) Hospital it seems necessary to include a short account of the stages by which this came about.

**Figure 7**. (facing page) The House of Industry - a ground floor plan in the 19th century. 1 Able-bodied Men's Day Room. 2 Cripple Ward Dormitory. 3 Cripple Ward. 4 Hall. 5 Old Men's Day Room. 6 Dining Room. 7 Porch. 8 Porter. 9 Board Room. 10 Master's Office. 11 Clerk's Office. 12 Bread Room. 13 Laundry. 14 Pump. 15 Wash-house. 16 East Ward 2. 17 East Ward 3. 18 East Ward 1, A.B. 19 Store. 20 Master's Pantry. 21 Master's Sitting Room. 22 Master's Kitchen. 23 Serve-out Passage. 24 Ovens. 25 Bakehouse. 26 Store. 27 Nursery Bedroom. 28 Nursery. 29 Old Women's Day Room. 30 Old Women's Dormitory. 31 Wash-house and bath. 32 Girls' Laundry and Scullery. 33 Girls' Day Room. 34 Girls' School Room. 35 Class Room. 36 Cottage. 37 Clerk's Sitting Room. 38 Sitting Room. 39 Band Room. 40 Kitchen. 41 Lavatories & Bath Room. 42 Boys' Dining Room. 43 Boys' School Room. 44 Males' Back Yard. 45 Males' Receiving Ward. 46 Males' Imbecile Ward. 47 Day Rooms. 48 Disinfecting Room. 49 Open Ward. 50 Wash House. 51 Drying Room. 52 Males' Kitchen. 53 Males' Lobby. 54 Staircase. 55 Male Attendant's Room. 56 Females' Kitchen. 57 Females' Lobby. 58 Staircase. 59 Female Attendant's Room. 60 Day Rooms. 61 Females' Back Yard. 62 W.C.s. 63 Female Imbecile Wards. 64 Bath Room. 65 Female Receiving Ward. 66 Kitchen. 67 Dining Room. 69 Urinal & W.C. 70 Open Shed. 71 A.B. Men's Yard. 72 Shoemaker's Shop. 73 Tailor's Shop. 74 General Store. 75 Store. 76,77,78,79,80 Open Yards. 81 Boiler House & Scullery. 82 Kitchen. 83,84 Open Yards. 85 Coke Yard. 86 Infants' Wash House & Store. 87 Coal Yard. 88 Smith's Shop. 89 Weighing Shed. 90 Bricklayer's Room. 91 W.C.s. 92 Girls' Playground. With acknowledgements and thanks to J. & J. Jones.

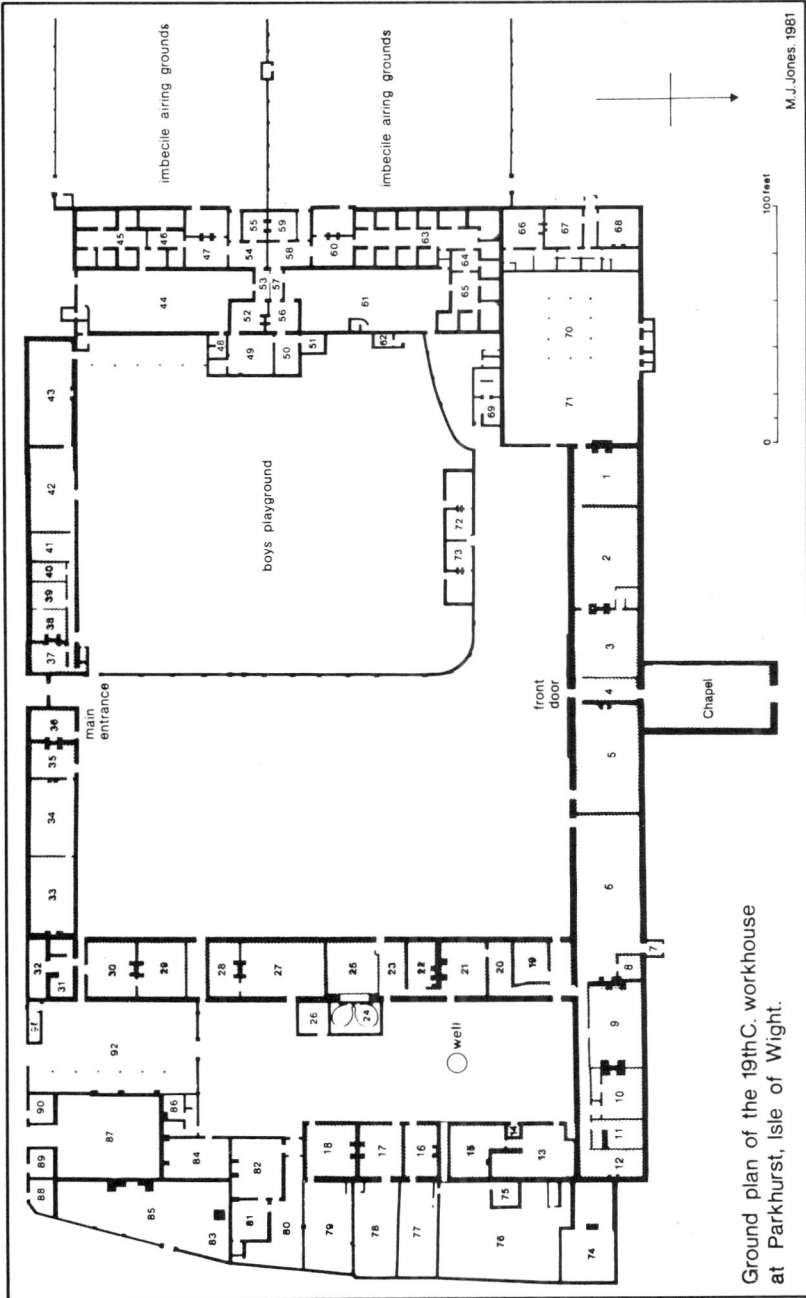

Ground plan of the 19thC. workhouse
at Parkhurst, Isle of Wight.

**Figure 7**

M.J.Jones. 1981

imbecile airing grounds

imbecile airing grounds

boys playground

main entrance

front door

Chapel

well

100 feet

81

The general plan given in the *Isle of Wight Illustrated History*, is of uncertain date, (see Fig. 7) but is some time in the later half of the 19th century; I am most grateful to Johanna Jones for the permission to reproduce this plan; it shows changes from the description given by Worsley, though at least on the ground floor, much of the original east/west main building with its chapel, and of the cross range, and of the set of rooms forming the east side of a smaller courtyard, remain more or less as they were, though with some change of usage. The south wing however has been converted into school rooms for girls on one side and boys on the other side of the gateway marked here as the main entrance; and it is on the west side, open in Worsley's days, that the big change has taken place; the wards for the mental defectives and the asylum filling up this side with a more or less continuous building and forming the fourth side of the quadrilateral. The large space so enclosed is divided into two; the larger incidentally shows a pattern of paths across what was presumably grass, this pattern being exactly the same as it was one hundred years later, before the day rooms which now divide the space were built. The smaller space, marked as the boys' playground, is separated from the larger by a wall, which is still there and still divides the two spaces; various later buildings now intrude into this smaller space. In the 1850s, £5 was spent on planting twelve lime trees around two sides of the boys' playground, these trees are shown in the Ordnance Survey Map of 1862; eleven pollarded limes are still there, and must I think be these very same trees.

All this is approximately the state shown in the Ordnance Survey Map based on the survey of 1862. (Fig. 4) It also shows the pond, somewhat larger and more rectangular than it was later; and a small pond, on the other (east) side of the path leading to the 'hospitals'; - it seems obvious that the drainage course of the large pond will have been through the smaller, and on, across or under Dodnor Lane through fields down to the river. The map also shows the two separate 'hospitals', the lower one (the 'Pest-house' of earlier days) with a small building at the north-east corner which must have been the mortuary added some years earlier, and the very small upper building near the top of the hill, - but obviously with some sort of clearing around it.

The map, (Fig. 5) based on a survey in 1940, shows many changes; the continuous building on the west side of the quadrilateral has given place to three separate buildings, - already mentioned - all still there today, - with modifications, and now known as Holly House, the Diabetic centre, and the secretary's cottage.

On the south side, part of the south wing labelled the girls' school room in previous maps, has gone, replaced by a wall, which itself was not brought down until the early 1970s. The buildings forming the east side of the smaller courtyard have been added to and altered; the 'Pest-house' is still there unchanged, but up the hill new buildings are seen. The small isolated building, - the former infectious diseases hospital has gone, - replaced by a mortuary. South of this are two small buildings: one had been the larger and later I.D. Hospital, and was now to become Bonchurch ward: the other was the Obstetric ward.

The larger buildings to the west of these three small ones are of course the Infirmary buildings, more or less as shown in Fig. 6, the whole group constituting Upper St. Mary's.

The Guardians in 1925 protested at a proposal that they should be abolished. However the writing was on the wall, and although they carried on for another five years their final meeting was on March 31st 1930; it was attended by about 60 members including 10 ladies. The Guardians had, if they are considered, despite administrative changes, to be the lineal descendants of the Directors of 1771, managed the House and its off-shoot the Infirmary and 'hospitals', for 160 years, latterly of course having many other functions on the Island, dealing with sewage and drainage, medical, nursing and maternity services, relief outside the Workhouse, schools and school attendance, rates, etc.

Their meetings were in the Sun Inn, Town Hall or in the Board Room of the Workhouse (their own printed forms continued to refer to it as the Workhouse right up to the end of their time); they had known controversy and dispute. They had included among their members aristocrats and landed gentry; retired service officers of high rank; learned professionals from medicine, the law, the church and teaching; merchants, farmers, craftsmen and tradesmen; ladies had been among the members for more than 30 years. Their quarterly and annual meetings sometimes numbered over 60, but quite often only half a dozen or fewer; once five members found themselves meeting on Christmas Day in the Sun Inn where meetings in those early years were sometimes held; they decided to postpone business for a week; once only a single member turned up (presumably with the clerk in attendance) he decided, one must suppose by a unanimous casting vote of one, to proceed. They had argued with the Poor Law Board and the later Local Government Board and had on occasions rejected and criticised their reports; once a distinguished Admiral had asked for an investigation into 'the mode of conducting business with a view to expediting proceedings...'. The Committee appointed reported its opinion that 'The business of the Board is conducted with as much dispatch as is consistent with due regard to accuracy; but that more time than is necessary is often taken up by desultory conversation'; - there is perhaps a message here for Committee chairmen - and members. In 1865, the year in which the Isle of Wight Corporation was dissolved, and the Isle of Wight Union created, they had decreed that their meetings should be held in public and that this should be made known to the press! In 1892 they had to get the consent of Winchester College for the improvement of the pathway leading from the hospital through the fields to Newport, - no objection was raised. In the same year they had protested to the Isle of Wight Central Railway at the inconvenience caused to members by the cancellation of the 9.40 train from Sandown to Newport; minutes do not reveal whether there was any response. In 1906 they wrote to the Royal Commission on Poor Law saying that the Commission should visit meetings of the Guardians around the country rather than merely hear evidence in London; and they supported a proposal by the Coventry Guardians that Ex-servicemen should be paid their pensions weekly instead of monthly, - that present practice being the source of thriftlessness and pauperism. (The Admiralty refused to make the change).

Now after their final meeting, closing with cheers for the chairman, Mr. H. Williams, they posed for a photograph and then proceeded to the Metropolitan Hall (later I am told Weeks Restaurant) had a farewell luncheon and sang 'Auld Lang Syne'.


Workhouses have acquired an evil name, and are often thought of and spoken of only in terms of bitter criticism and condemnation; the sordid and sometimes cruel conditions in which paupers and children were kept in them were perhaps due in part to deliberate governmental intent to make them as unattractive as possible, in part through sheer bureaucracy and bumbledom; and in part to simple lack of interest or knowledge. It seems that the House of Industry had its bad times, - as in 1813, 40 years after its foundation, when enquiries revealed many shortcomings and malpractices, and the Master was required to resign (in the report the 'medical gentlemen' were specifically absolved of any impropriety or failure in their duties); and much later than that Bill Shepard has written of distressing cruelties to children in Newport. Nevertheless, the House of Industry was unusual in that it was founded not by Order of the Government, but by the initiative of a group of local inhabitants who assumed the management of it; and when after some 60 years, it came under the control first of the Poor Law Board, and later of the Local Government Board, the Guardians who in effect ran it, were local men and the management was handed down through the generations from those who first took it on collectively and, especially in the early years, they must have known personally many of those who had to find refuge in the House.

Small may or may not be beautiful, but it does afford a degree of personal knowledge, interest, and understanding which become diluted as numbers and size increase. It seems apparent that over the years the Directors and Guardians had a genuine concern for the inmates and many matters were agreed and directions given for promoting their relative comfort and well-being, the education and training of the children, and the care of the sick and disabled.

In June 1789 it was decided that all disabled boys might be apprenticed to the Governor of the House of Industry, to learn weaving until the age of 18, and after discharge should be provided with looms at the expense of the Corporation and with materials and employment to exercise their trade, being paid at the usual rate for goods delivered to the House of Industry. It was a long time before a ladies committee was elected who were to visit the House of Industry; so early as 1834 it was thought that 'Great good might result from the attendance of a committee of ladies ... under the control of the chaplain', - but it was not until 1895 under the chairmanship of P. Glynn Esq. that such a committee came into being.

There was an endeavour to provide games and amusements for the children; in 1853 swings in the girls' yard were made safe, and a year later there was reference to a racquet or fives court in the boys' yard. Pocket handkerchiefs were provided for children in 1856, and rice with treacle was to take the place of pea soup which was not well liked; at that time also cod liver oil was found to be a medicine not a food. Simple games, toys, balls and illustrated journals were sought for the idiot wards. The Mayor of Newport invited children at the House of Industry to the celebrations at the Wedding of the Prince of Wales, - the Governor thanked him and also Mr. Charles Newnham, Confectioner, for his kindness. In 1860 a mast was erected in the boys' yard, by Messrs White of Cowes, - with a £10 donation towards it from the Rev. McAlb, the Chaplain. Boys were to have musical instruction in 1871 and four guineas was made available for the purchase of fifes and drums. In 1895 a special allowance of £35 per annum was granted for a blind boy to enable him to study at the Royal National College at Norwood and the Academy of Music, and in 1901 the college wrote thanking the Board for their help in this case and saying that the boy now had a certificate in piano tuning. (Almost a century later Tina Snow who is typing the script of this book for me was trained in the same institute, now known as the Royal National College for the Blind). The care of the deaf and dumb was a matter of concern and difficulty and there were repeated enquiries about accommodation in the mainland institute for such sufferers. In

1877 books were received from the Seely Library and in 1880 adult classes in reading, writing and arithmetic were started for men living in the House of Industry; classes for women were to follow, - one hour daily in the evenings (not Saturdays); in 1888 there was reference to the Workhouse library; a concert was offered and accepted; and the next year the circulation of *Warcry*, the journal of the Salvation Army, was allowed; in 1891 Miss Elgar played the harmonium and taught children singing.

On a number of occasions such as Royal weddings and coronations roast beef and plum pudding were served; very nice when they happened to fall in the cool half of the year, - but perhaps rather lacking in imagination at the Golden Jubilee in 1887 on Mid Summer's Day; but not ungenerous - in 1863, for the Prince of Wales's wedding, minutes record the supply of thirty score of beef, three score of suet, and 95lb each of currants and raisins! In 1892 came a letter from the new County Council about the establishment of a School of Horticulture, which after several exchanges went ahead.

These few extracts from the minutes and others, reveal I believe that the history of the House of Industry was not one of unremitting hardship and a total lack of consideration or humanity. My wife recalls talking to an old lady in the 1960s, who remembered how she used to visit her aunt in the Workhouse before the First World War, and how on Saturday afternoons, in the winter, the old ladies would sit round a fire having hot scones for their tea with a white tablecloth. On the other hand Miss Weedon recalls how in 1947 the mentally defective girls living in what is now Holly House were marched to the laundry, worked there during the day and were marched back again at five o'clock, fed and locked into their rooms till the next morning. There are two sides to every story.

After County Council took over the House and the Infirmary there were a number of important developments. During this phase of the hospital's life, management was delegated mainly to the Public Assistance Committee and its sub-committees; they made recommendations to the council and supervised the building and works that were ordered. The County Medical Officer reported to the Health (and Housing) Committee, and had some overall authority for the staffing and management of the hospital, as well of course as for the Health Service run by the council outside the hospital. The Master of the House of Industry remained responsible for the day to day maintenance within the Infirmary, but the medical and nursing work of the hospital was in the hands of the Superintendent Nurse and the appointed Medical Officer, namely Dr G. Raymond who worked part-time at the Infirmary for the council from 1930 to 1937, when he retired, and was followed by Dr Clement Sylvester who was joined in 1939 by Dr Peskett as his deputy.

It was the Public Assistance Committee (P.A.C.) that decided in 1935 to rename the Infirmary St. Mary's Hospital; St. Luke and St. Faith had been considered as alternatives and in Newport one might have expected St. Thomas, St. James or St. Cross to be considered, but St. Mary's was decided upon possibly from the association with Carisbrooke Parish and the Church of St. Mary's there. The change of name was approved by the Registrar General - reported in January 1936. At about the same time a brass plate was placed at the entrance to the House of Industry confirming the name Forest House.

The number of residents in the combined House and Infirmary during the 1930s varied between 300 and 350; of these there were usually around 120 in the Infirmary, - about 50 men and 70 women, - the beds for women including ten for maternity cases; the House usually held rather less than 200, - in the so-called 'Ordinary Wards'; and there were about 40 in the wards for mental defectives; the care of this last group was shared between the part-time Medical Officer to the Infirmary and a Medical Superintendent at Whitecroft.

In 1934 it was recorded that an agreement had been reached between the County Hospital and St. Mary's; the former would take all 'acute and sub acute cases', and the Infirmary would accommodate the chronic cases.

This book is not the place in which to enter into a discussion of such terms; the word chronic has been misunderstood and misused by the laity and ultimately, at times anyhow, by both medical and nursing professions; and above all by the media and finally dare one say it, by the powers that be; it has been thought of and used at times as indicating the severity of an illness or disability, and has even tended, too often, to become a term expressing contempt or abuse without actually uttering it. What was implied at this stage was that patients with chronic disabilities or illnesses were not expected to recover and often not to be discharged from hospital; and at the same time they were not thought likely to benefit from the attention of any medical or surgical consultant or the treatment they could offer; so that the wards for the chronically sick or disabled patients were filled by those who usually remained for a long time, often to their lives end; no doubt there were exceptions. Some recovered sufficiently to be considered no longer in need of nursing and medical attention. Such patients who had been admitted by the P.A.C. often perhaps from the Workhouse itself, and usually unable to support themselves, could be transferred to the Workhouse. This raised other problems.

On the one hand the doctors were repeatedly asserting that there was always a demand for beds in the Infirmary, and hence always the need to discharge any patient who was fit to live elsewhere; on the other hand, as the Committee pleaded, while hospital patients continued to draw their Old Age Pension, once they were transferred to the Workhouse this ceased; some members of the Committee felt strongly that old people were being treated unfairly by such transfers; a possible solution was found in the use of the sick wards in the House of Industry; patients placed in these wards could be regarded as receiving hospital care; and as early as 1931 the appointment of a night attendant for the old ladies in the House of Industry, would it was thought, justify the transfer of at least two or three patients from the Infirmary to the House. The matter however remained controversial and disagreement persisted and at times perhaps became heated. Eventually in 1941, Mr. Phillips, a General Inspector of the Ministry of Health was asked to consider and report; and he seems to have achieved an oracular judgement, as might be expected of a high civil servant, saying that it was the doctors' sole prerogative to decide whether a patient required medical or surgical treatment, but it was the job of the Master of the House in accordance with his Committee's instructions to decide whether any particular individual should be accommodated in the hospital or transferred to the Workhouse; he added that he believed that borderline cases, - where there was an element of doubt, should stay in hospital; and, most importantly, that medical and surgical treatment did not include nursing care. That is, - patients or residents of the House who did not need medical or surgical treatment, might nevertheless need the services of the nursing staff. Dr Sylvester, for his part, assured the Inspector and the Committee that he had never given instructions for the transfer of patients, he had merely recommended the Master to do so. After this judgement a lay sub-committee was appointed to decide upon transfer from hospital to House in each individual case!

Work was needed during these years on the accommodation of nurses and a kitchen and staff dining room in the Infirmary; on the provision for mental defectives; on the porter's lodge and reception rooms associated with it; and on the obstetric accommodation. All the building during this next decade was contracted for by J. Ball & Sons.

The first of the items to be dealt with was the Infirmary kitchen which was remodelled and supplied with two Esse stoves. Lacking any plans it is difficult to judge precisely how the original buildings were designed and how they were now changed and extended. There was at first a scheme to build a new nurses home on the west side of the drive and in front of (i.e below) the Infirmary; it would have been roughly on the site of the short-lived chapel built in the 1960s and demolished in the 1980s when the new St. Mary's was built; however this plan never got off the ground and additional rooms for nurses were provided over the extended north wing of the central administrative block to which dining rooms and sitting-rooms for nurses and sisters were added as well as the remodelled kitchen. Some rooms had already been put on the upper floors of this block in 1910 and more were now added, the minutes indicating that they were reached by a corridor through the older rooms. The new block was opened by Sir Godfrey Baring in 1935 and was named the Eva Baring Wing; it provided about 20 bedrooms for nurses; it was centrally heated and lighted by electricity.

Plans for a new maternity ward were considered about the same time in 1931; at the start it was suggested that two 'pavilions' should be built, - one to be kept for infectious or septic cases; however Dr Fairley recommended that such infectious cases should be treated at Fairlee Hospital, and that one pavilion would suffice. The initial plan submitted by the County Surveyor in July 1931 was estimated to cost £4,000, and the building sub-committee, taken aback at this expense, recommended the rejection of the plan to the P.A.C. However, this Committee accepted it and recommended the County Council to seek a loan of £4,000. The building, separate at the start from the rest of the hospital, was completed in 1933; the electricity supply was obtained by a connection to the cable supplying Albany Barracks, and involved a payment of £3-2s-5d for connecting up and 8d per unit, to the War Department. The final account for this pavilion was paid in October 1933 and it was completed before the work on the new nurses home was finished. The P.A.C. decreed that the new pavilion was in the first place provided for 'necessitous cases', i.e. for women who could not afford care at home or in any of the available maternity homes or had no home; complicated and abnormal midwifery cases came next in priority; others only if room was available. The pavilion was built on the site of a tennis court that had been available for nurses and a new court was provided in its place and must be the one still present in front of what later became known as Nurses Home Two.

The new mortuary, planned in 1933, was built in 1934 on the site of the small old building used first for infectious diseases and known at this time to hospital workers as the Smallpox Hospital, - although it had been many years since sufferers from Smallpox had been admitted, and the Smallpox Hospital at Ashey had been available since about the end of the First World War. The demolition of this old building had been ordered in 1931.

In 1934-35 joint meetings of the committees dealing with accommodation for the mentally defective patients and with works and buildings, a sub-committee of the P.A.C., agreed that provision for these patients should be continued at Parkhurst rather than at Whitecroft, unless any better accommodation became available, and that it should be increased to about 100 beds, either in the existing buildings, modified, or in new buildings; and in August 1935 a draft plan was submitted for a new block for male mentally deficient patients to house 54 patients and to include two large day rooms and a work room. Two years later the committee for mentally defective patients were considering the appropriation of 30 acres of land north-east of St. Mary's on which to establish a colony for mental defectives; the land however was found unsuitable, and consideration was given to forming such a colony at the Hermitage, or at North Court! In the following year a plan for the temporary use of a house, Woodside, in Pallance Road, Northwood was produced, - which inevitably led to protest from the local resident population.

The building opposite the Forest Road which had been put up in 1895, had housed the porter's lodge and reception wards and had been for some 40 years at the main entrance to the hospital; now it was found to be in poor repair and unsafe; some rooms had been closed. In the next year the Works and Buildings Committee planned a new lodge with a weighbridge at the entrance; it was to provide also a flat for a married man above the lodge and was to be at the new main entrance to the hospital. A row of buildings running up along the drive from it were to provide admission wards, one two bedded ward, and one single ward, for both men and women with bathroom, WC and linen store; this building was completed just after the outbreak of war. The old building was used for a time as a store, later it was suggested that it could be a cleansing station (?decontamination centre) and later an accessory fire station with a fire engine garaged close by; finally it was renovated and in part provided a residence for the newly appointed head gardener and his family immediately after the war. More changes would come later.

In 1933 the P.A.C. considered 'a small operating room for emergencies'; but it was only in 1937 that the provision of an operating theatre was reconsidered and the theatre installed at the Borstal Institute (Camphill) was inspected; and the next year the P.A.C. agreed to a new maternity ward of four beds; a labour ward and nursery, operating room and wards for eight children and eleven women. However any action on this was postponed partly because of the indeterminate status of the hospital, and partly because of the expectation of a conference with other Island hospitals and the Public Health Committee. Also postponed was the repair of the covered ways between the central administrative blocks and the male and female wards on either side, - those covered ways which as J. & J. Jones wrote had been the object of dispute between the Guardians and the L.G.B. half a century earlier.

Early in the war or in the months just before it the C.M.O. reported that the Ministry supported a plan for an operating theatre; however soon after that in October 1939 they dropped plans for upgrading the hospital and further work was again delayed; and the Classification Committee rejected a suggestion that the hospital should be renamed (again) ' St. Mary's Emergency Hospital', - on the grounds that it had not been upgraded. The possibility of a theatre remained however, and the Chairman of the P.A.C. inspected an operating table offered for £12; an Occupational Therapist, Miss Thirkell, was appointed for two sessions each of five hours weekly (4s an hour + lunch and tea).

At last in 1942 plans for an operating theatre and for conversion of the infectious disease wards for use associated with the surgical work, and for an X-ray room, were adopted, - it was said that the Ministry would pay 70%, - and by July 1942 it was reported that the theatre would be ready in about two weeks; a Sister was appointed for the theatre and the surgical ward; and the next year improvements were made in the sterilising and anaesthetic rooms and in the associated ward, and a covered way about 100ft. long was built leading from the ladies end of the main hospital to the theatre, etc.; this building work was undertaken by G.H. Williams of Wootton.

The services of the hospital had been improved in other ways during the 1930s. In September 1933 the Newport Co-operative offered water at 6d per thousand gallons which the Infirmary accepted. Central heating was improved and fire escapes provided for the wards. Electric lighting for the Infirmary was recommended in 1934 and for the House in 1937; certainly new buildings were provided with electric light and at some stage the rest of the Infirmary, but years later the Superintendent Nurse was complaining of the poor lighting in some of the E.M.S. wards which she said were still only illuminated by paraffin lamps.

During these years while the P.A.C. was in charge of the hospital and the House as a whole the C.M.O., Dr Fairley, reported to the Public Health Committee on matters of nursing staff and training and on questions of infectious diseases and midwifery services. Admission to the hospital which had hitherto been authorised only by the P.A.C. could after 1935 or so be arranged through the Public Health Committee; the significance of this, one supposes, was that admissions were to be made now not only on the basis of poverty and the need for assistance from the council, but also on the count simply of medical or surgical necessity; that is the Infirmary was becoming more of a hospital rather than just an appendix to the Workhouse.

Dr Fairley in 1937 reported on the training of nurses; lectures for nurses as mentioned, had been provided earlier at St. Mary's, but had been abandoned in 1921, since the Infirmary was not recognised as a training school, and because, unfortunately, such a large proportion of nurses in those earlier years had not remained in the hospital long enough to complete any sort of training; many of them came and went over a period of a few months or a year. He advised a joint arrangement with the County Hospital and Fairlee Hospital for the training of nurses; tuition should be provided for nurses at St. Mary's and also at the Frank James Hospital and at the two Shanklin hospitals (Scio House and the Arthur Webster Hospital); training at Whitecroft and at the Royal National Hospital he considered satisfactory.

By 1940 the numbers of nursing staff had increased; besides the Superintendent Nurse (who it was specified later in 1946 should not be referred to as Matron, a term reserved for the Matron of the House) there were 5 sisters, 6 staff nurses and 25 assistant nurses; there were also 6 resident maids and 6 non-resident ward maids; 1 cook and 1 assistant cook and 1 kitchen maid; and 1 ambulance driver and handyman.

A new set of 38 rules for nurses was issued; the first was that nurses must obey all directions from the Superintendent Nurse and the Medical Officer; the 38th was that all bedroom doors were to be kept locked.

Further additions to the staff were made, - including of course those mentioned when the theatre and related buildings were opened. There was however a continuing shortage of accommodation for nurses and difficulty in war-time in recruiting the necessary staff; it is mentioned that in 1942 ten nurses were provided by local nursing associations and were presumably non-resident.

Dr Sylvester and Dr Peskett continued as Medical Officers, but the start of surgery required additional appointments and in May 1943, Mr. Leisching was appointed Visiting Surgeon for P.A.C. patients; also in 1942 when the X-ray room was built in association with the theatre, Dr E.G. Barker was appointed part-time radiologist. The X-ray apparatus unfortunately gave a good deal of trouble and was often out of order for months on end, and during this time the House Governor at Osborne House agreed to the use of their apparatus for which the Committee was duly grateful.

In the House of Industry the chapel was part of the original building, and more or less unchanged for 150 years, and the Chaplain had been one of the resident staff; but soon both chapel and chaplaincy must change. In 1938 the Works and Buildings Sub Committee suggested that the gallery of the chapel should be boarded up, and the chapel itself redecorated; this however had to stand over for the time being and was again postponed in 1939; and in 1940, presumably under the stress of war and the increased activity in the hospital and the House as a whole, the Committee agreed to the use of the chapel as a store for civil defence equipment. (I have not found any mention of its deconsecration). Thereafter services were held in the Board room, and the chapel a few years later became known to hospital workers as 'Knocker's Store', - 'Knocker' White being in charge of the stores, - and the nickname differentiating him from 'Deffy White', the Engineer who was hard of hearing.

The Chaplain had since the 1890s lived in one of the three buildings on the west side of the House; it had needed fairly frequent repair and alteration; the Chaplain besides his hospital work in the 1930s did some teaching at Cowes and Sandown, one supposes that his income was thereby supplemented. He seems to have been in a subordinate position to the Master, who in 1930 rejected his request for an issue of 50 hymn books, without apparently any reference to the Committee. There was a suggestion now that the Resident Chaplain should be replaced by a part-time Visiting Chaplain; the Committee thought that simple corporate prayers might be read morning and evening; attendance should be encouraged (but presumably was not compulsory), and committee members should attend divine service from time to time.

The Rev. Bayliss who had been Chaplain for several years died in 1937 and in 1938 the Rev. Kelsey was appointed a part-time Non-resident Chaplain. The Chaplain's house, - referred to in the minutes on one occasion as the 'old parsonage', became a few years later the Master's house. This was after Mr. McKeown, Master, had retired in 1945 with the thanks and good wishes of the management. Mr. Bennett was appointed in his place; he evidently found the house in poor repair and ordered some work to be done on it which brought him into dispute with his Committee, whose authority he had not asked for; for this reason and others they would have dismissed him, but refrained because of his hitherto unblemished record and for the need to obtain the Minister's consent for taking such a step; so he remained and was still in post when the N.H.S. took over. Apart from becoming the venue for religious services, the Boardroom also now was to serve as a cinema; in 1937 the decision was taken to install a cinematograph projector and a projection room was made at the back of the Board room; the equipment was paid for by public subscription. Also in 1937, Messrs Sherratts provided six portable wireless sets for the wards, - for £50, with full guarantees, 'including valve replacements'. New laundry equipment was also installed in the House during this decade.

At a meeting of the Public Assistance Committee which must have been one of the last, if not the very last, at which the Committee concerned itself with the affairs of St. Mary's, the fate of some furniture and utensils at the H of I was considered; 12 Chippendale chairs were to go to the office of the Superintendent Registrar; a mahogany desk to the ladies' room in County Hall; and four pewter plates and two silver spoons were to be placed in the County Hall; all of these as 'a memorial to the work of the Poor Law Administration now being wound up'.

# IV

# WHITECROFT HOSPITAL

When the Isle of Wight became a separate county in 1890, it ceased to have any proprietary rights in the Hampshire County Mental Hospital at Knowle; Isle of Wight patients such as were already there remained there for the time being, and others were sent; but the county had to pay for each patient, the fee decided by the Hampshire county, and it was known that Knowle Hospital was already overcrowded, and Hampshire county was anxious to take over the accommodation used by the Isle of Wight; some Isle of Wight patients of course were at the House of Industry as has already been explained.

A meeting was held in Newport Guild Hall on March 2nd 1892, Gen. the Right. Hon. Somerset I.G. Calthorpe, Chairman of the County Council presided; to consider establishing a mental hospital on the Island.

The first step was to get land; the Commission in Lunacy, - a national body, - had let it be known that about 50 acres would be required. They had enquired first of the Guardians of the possibility of purchasing land on the House of Industry site; but nothing came of this and other offers were invited. It is perhaps rather remarkable that no less than about a dozen different farms offered that amount of land, - including those at Parkhurst, Furzyhurst, Marvel, Longdown, Hale, Redway, Great and Little Pan, Merstone, Rookley Waightshale, Stoneshill and Whitecroft: after the committee had considered all these, the Commissioners in Lunacy were asked to look at two of them, Redway and Whitecroft; it was reckoned that accommodation would be needed for 250 'paupers' and for 30 private (paying) patients; and an administrative block, making a total population of 350. In August 1893, the Redway site was eliminated and in October the Whitecroft site was approved, on condition that it should also include the field known as Peddars Butts; the Bursar of Winchester College agreed to sell this latter for £650.

Architects were then invited to submit plans for buildings; a block system was required, each block to accommodate 50 patients and to be of two storeys; there was to be a laundry and administrative block to include accommodation for a Superintendent and for an unmarried Medical Officer; a dining hall for 200; six cottages for attendants; and later a chapel. A water tower would be needed and the wards and buildings were to be fitted for electric light. The

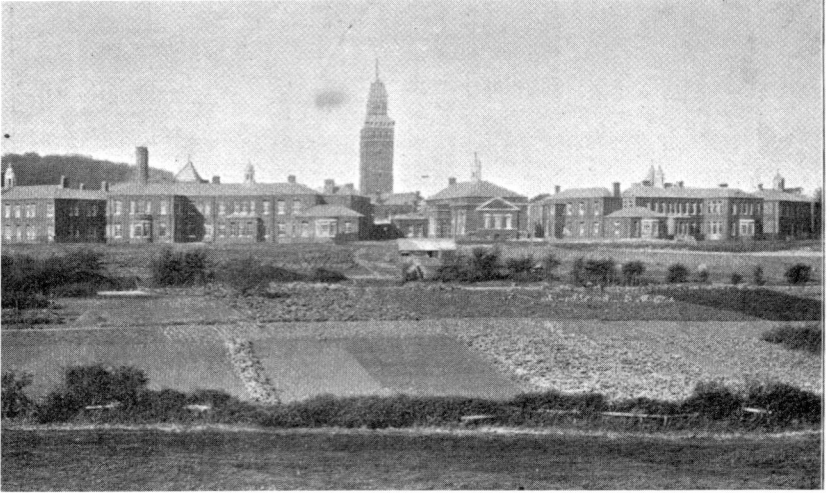

**Plate 8**. Whitecroft Hospital. An early view from the south-east, before the nurses' home was built. *Courtesy: R.G. McInnes.*

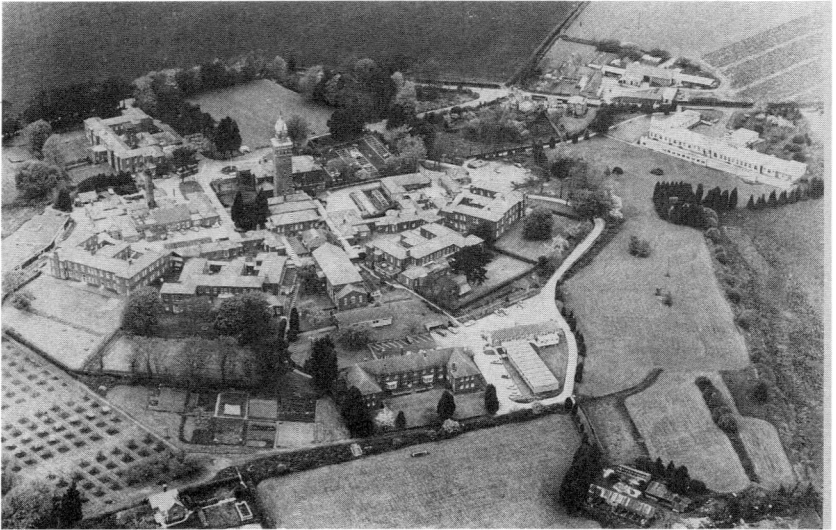

**Plate 9**. An aerial view of Whitecroft Hospital. Thompson House is on the right. The two main entrances can be seen; and Tennyson Ward at the side of the drive leading up to the central buildings and clock tower. The Occupational Therapy building and the laundry are to the left of this. *Courtesy: Mr. J. Lewis (& others?).*

winning design would carry with it the contract for the buildings; second, third and fourth prizes of £50, £30 and £20 were to be awarded for the runners up.

A visit was paid to the Hants County Mental Hospital at Knowle about this time. It had 461 men and 529 women patients, of this 69 men and 103 women were Islanders and chargeable to the Isle of Wight. Soon after this, the Hampshire County Council informed the Isle of Wight that their asylum was seriously overcrowded, and they hoped the Isle of Wight asylum would be ready for occupation in 1894; also that they were building a new block for idiot children, and would charge the Island two elevenths of the price of this.

After much consideration and correspondence, Mr. G.H. Howell was appointed to judge the plans and designs submitted, and he selected those of Mr. B. Jacobs of East Yorkshire. Controversy arose over the selection of the plans and the award of the contract. Before the building was even started a Visiting Committee was selected and appointed; the need and propriety of this was questioned and a legal opinion (given by Mr. Edward Bullen at some length) was that an asylum must by law have a Visiting Committee, - but a Visiting Committee was not obliged to have an asylum and would therefore properly be appointed in advance of the building. The land purchased was in excess of needs and the surplus was sold off to Mr. Ford at £1 an acre after his offer of ten shillings an acre had been declined.

Messrs Garlick and Horton of 43 Sloane Street, SW were the builders; bricks were made on site, - three and a half million of them; Swanage stone was to be used, but when it was not available Bath stone was accepted instead, albeit after much debate. A heating installation, by Henry Hope of Birmingham, cost £1,212 and an electric lighting plant, with its own generator, by Sheddon of Southampton cost £2,453. A clock with two dials and a ten hundred weight bell was supplied by John Smith. This clock, high up in the tower, was, and is, visible over a considerable extent of the Island: and the saying that someone is 'Under the Clock' as a euphemism for being in the Mental Hospital, has been familiar on the Island through this century.

Building proceeded slowly. It started early in 1894, - one report says in February, but the contract with the builder was sealed only on April 27th; in June 1895 it was reported that work had been delayed by four and a half months by inclement weather, by workman strikes, by shortage of workers, and by a fever epidemic; also the isolated position of the work was unpopular. Water supply became a problem. Newport Corporation had at the start offered ten thousand gallons a day subject to terms; but it was decided to sink a well and this was done to a depth of 74ft. with a bore hole below that to an additional 100ft.

The plans as agreed were to include a block for the sick and infirm; one for recent and acute cases; and one for epileptics; each of these three were to house 29 men and 41 women, a total of 210; a fourth block was to be for working, quiet and chronic patients with room for 13 men and 17 women, bringing the total to 240; it was anticipated that a further two blocks, each perhaps with accommodation for 55 patients, would raise the total to 350. In addition there were to be farm buildings, a cemetery and a mortuary.

Whitecroft Hospital thus differed from Ryde and St. Mary's in that it opened with most of its accommodation already nearly built and its final shape and plan more or less settled. Besides this, the staff were to be appointed by the time the hospital opened and it would be some time before there were any substantial changes in the staffing.

Knowle Hospital may surely be fairly looked upon as the parent of Whitecroft; the buildings of Whitecroft copied many features of those at Knowle; the first medical Superintendent appointed had been a Medical Officer at Knowle for some years before coming to Whitecroft and came direct from there; not only so, but both the head male and female attendants came from Knowle and so of course did many of the first batch of patients.

The hospital, although large by Island standards, was much smaller than many of the county asylums and because of this, the head male and female attendants, each of whom received £50 a year salary, living in, had to include in their duties those of the House Keeper, supervisor of the cooking, and in the case of the man, the work of patients employed in the workshops; he was also required to have a knowledge of music. Carpenters, tailors and fitters workshops were furnished before the hospital opened. Other staff besides these senior attendants included, for 80 men, three charge attendants, five under-attendants, and two night-attendants, their salaries being about £30 a year each with the charge attendants slightly higher; and for 120 ladies, four charge nurses at £20 to £22 a year, two night-nurses at the same salary and eight under-nurses at £17 to £20 a year. There was one laundry maid, three kitchen maids and one house maid. Attendants and nurses who held the Certificate of the Medico-Psychological Association were granted £1 a year extra. The cook had £25 to £30 a year and for the asylum band there was an allowance of £20 a year and uniforms. All staff of course lived in, and there was an allowance of £40 annually for books, papers, amusements and periodicals. The total cost of furnishing the hospital before it opened was £3,000.

Dr H. Shaw M.B. D.P.H. was the first Medical Superintendent; coming from Knowle he was appointed in August 1895 and actually started in September 1896; he had a salary of £350 with 'the usual allowances', living in; these would one supposes have included accommodation for himself and later for his family, possibly a board allowance, heating, lighting and some domestic assistance. He was authorised in February 1896 to appoint and discharge the hospital servants.

Workers in the Engineering Department and stokers, living in, received respectively tuppence and a penny a day.

There was no formal opening ceremony. The chairman of the County Council explained that he did not think such a ceremony appropriate.

Soon after the opening a private patient block was available with a billiard room. This was the block near the main gate separate from the rest of the hospital; later it became an admission ward, and was named Tennyson Ward.

The post of Assistant Medical Officer was advertised in June 1896 and was soon filled by Dr B. Taafe Trim who received £100 a year and all found, except for alcoholic drinks.

40 male patients, it is recorded, were transferred from Knowle on July 7th 1896, but temporary difficulties in water supply at the hospital and trouble in the crossing from Stokes Bay led to postponement of further transfers until September. The available accommodation was in excess of needs, and patients were accepted from other councils - 30 from the LCC and 8 from West Sussex. At the end of the first year there were 220 patients, the numbers increased steadily and after another year there were 304.

In the first Annual Report by the Medical Superintendent, he indicated that a block to hold 50 private patients would soon be ready, and that a lodge, farm buildings and two cottages were under construction. Male patients worked on the land; two had 'escaped' but were soon brought back; there were weekly dances and occasional concerts. The cost per patient was twelve shillings weekly; this cost was actually to decline during the next few years to as low as ten shillings and threepence weekly. The accounts for the first year showed:-

| | |
|---|---|
| Salaries for officers | £570 |
| Wages for attendants and others | £563 |
| Provisions | £1351 |
| Gas and water | £855 |
| Surgery and dispensary | £27 |

There was a deficit of £26 on the farm in the first year. One may note the low expenditure on alcoholic drinks, especially compared with, for example, the County Hospital and St. Mary's. The Commissioners had been pleased to learn that extended exercise beyond the grounds was afforded to the patients twice weekly weather permitting.

The water supply was a continuing problem in these early years and was considered to be linked to the two cases of Typhoid Fever in the year 1896-97; a new well had been dug and two years later a bore hole had been driven down to 400ft. and later as deep as 525ft., which was found to suffice. At an early stage too a new boiler was required which weighed twenty tons, and must have provided a formidable problem for transport along the local highways; and soon the electricity installation failed and another £750 had to be spent on it, but it still gave further trouble. The commissioners had asked for improved safety precautions, and implied the need for a chapel. The number of out-county patients, i.e., patients from the mainland, reached 81 during this year. It was a number which varied considerably, declining from this high level to no more than three in the years just before the war, but rising again after the end of the First World War. The charge for county patients at this stage was twelve shillings and threepence weekly and for out-county patients fourteen shillings; private patients whether Isle of Wight or mainland paid twenty-five shillings.

Visits were paid in these early years by deputations from the Boards of Governors of several other unions including those of Wandsworth and Clapham, and also by the B.M.A. during a meeting in Portsmouth, and all of these generally approved of the hospital. It was noted that no restraint was used and only one patient was sedated.

The classification of mental diseases at this time is shown in the figures for 1899 of patients in the hospital:-

| Type of Illness | Male | Female | Total |
|---|---|---|---|
| Congenital | 3 | 2 | 5 |
| Epilepsy | 8 | 3 | 11 |
| G.P.I. | 5 | 1 | 6 |
| Mania | 49 | 93 | 142 |
| Melancholia | 7 | 29 | 36 |
| Dementia | 31 | 60 | 91 |
| Total | 103 | 188 | 291 |

During these early years, and indeed for a long time thereafter, the farm, - in which some of the male residents worked - produced meat, poultry, eggs and vegetables in some quantity.

The Commissioners in lunacy paid yearly visits and made reports, -

sometimes a bit critical; thus in their report for 1904 they wrote 'We think it would be as well to encourage the male attendants to produce a general tidier appearance' and in 1913 they recommended an improvement in diet, - there should be a second (pudding) course at the main meal; a better allowance of meat in soup and pies, currently 2oz, and sometimes a cake for tea.

In the first year of the war Dr Shaw died; he had been at Whitecroft for nearly 20 years; he had married a few years earlier, I think in 1905. It was clear from the minutes that as Medical Superintendent he was very definitely in charge of the hospital, and answerable to the committee for all aspects of it; and one gets the impression that he was competent to manage it and had the trust and goodwill of the Committee.

Dr Peachell followed him but stayed for only about a year, moving to Dorset; the committee had declined to liberate him for enlistment, but had required him to decide how many male staff could be spared to join the forces.

He was followed by Dr Erskine who was to receive £400 a year rising to £500 by increments of £25 yearly; he also had his house, lighting, upkeep of the garden, and the privilege of purchasing from the hospital stores, worth £100; and he also received £50 a year as Medical Officer to the Mental Deficiency Committee. It was decided that he and his assistant were to have a month's holiday each during the year; there would be no locum tenens, but local practitioners would be asked to relieve. Later in the war, presumably when manpower was becoming a problem, the Board of Control suggested that one Medical Officer was sufficient and the Assistant, Dr Reardon, was allowed to go and work in another asylum, his wife being authorised to stay in her lodgings at Whitecroft. In 1917 the nurses appealed for one whole day a week off duty, but the Committee decided that this would have to wait until the end of the war.

In January 1919 there were 380 patients in the hospital, this number included 58 private patients; 38 'out-county' patients; and 7 service patients; most of the 'out-county' patients returned during the year to Portsmouth or Chichester and only one remained after that.

The Medical Superintendent reported in 1921 that there had been three cases of Typhoid Fever; one healthy infant had been born; four patients had escaped and been recaptured; he referred to the recommendations of the Conciliation Joint Committee of Mental Hospital Associates and National asylum workers; there had been agreement upon a 60 hour working week (five days of 12 hours and two days off each week) and some rise in weekly wages.

As Medical Officer to the Mental Deficiency Committee, the Superintendent reported difficulty in finding vacancies for the most severely afflicted mental defectives; they had to go either to a suitable guardian or to an asylum; he visited these cases, accompanied by the senior female attendant.

During 1919, 445 patients received treatment; 380 had been on the register on January 1st and 65 had been admitted; 75 were discharged; and 44 died; of the 324 remaining, only 56 were over 65.

The annual reports indicate a steady evolution of the hospital; patients were allowed out with friends at weekends, or were taken out by the staff; the kitchens were improved; the hospital was recognised as a training school for female and male nurses and a Sister Tutor was appointed; the staff had been increased - there were by 1925 five male charge nurses and 13 male attendants, six female charge nurses and 29 other nurses, and 10 nurses were certified as Registered Mental Nurses.

Occupational classes had been started, directed by women under the Matron; the women taught handiwork such as raffia work, cane tray making, basket making and knitting. Men as before worked on the farm or in the tailor's or carpenter's shop or the Engineering Department. It was hoped to start an occupational class for men soon. In this year the total cost of wages and salaries was £8,150 and of provisions £4,580. The hospital kitchens had been improved and all food for private patients was now cooked in these kitchens, not in separate kitchens in the private block; but a deputation from the Board of Guardians complained that the food there in the private block was never hot and advised some system of keeping it hot. The hospital now was overcrowded to the extent of 24 patients.

Throughout the late 1920s accommodation for mental defectives was a continual problem; Portsmouth and Southampton had been approached, but were unable to help; 10 cases were under supervision at the Brighton Guardianship Society, and 34 were at home under supervision, visited by Medical Officer and nurse; there were 26 patients at Parkhurst and 15 in institutions elsewhere, but such institutions would no longer be able to take new cases.

In 1930 there is mention of the Mental Deficiency Act which was said to indicate an expectation of 8 mental defectives per thousand population; at that time this would have given a total of 752 for the Island; the number ascertained was 195; the accommodation needed on the Island, reckoned at one per thousand population, would be 94; in fact it was 64. Of all those on the Island 41 were in institutions, 45 were under supervision, 11 under guardianship, 24 under voluntary supervision, 38 now at Parkhurst, i.e. St. Mary's and 16 at Whitecroft, but suitable for institutions which could give day and night care.

Dr Erskine had been Medical Superintendent from 1915 to 1932 and now he retired and his place was taken by Dr Charles Davies-Jones who came from Oxfordshire and a year later was joined by Dr A. Wood. It was at this stage that Whitecroft Hospital became known as a Mental Hospital and no longer as a Lunatic Asylum. Some out-patient work had already been established by Dr Erskine, who visited and advised on patients with General Practitioners; soon after he came, Dr Davies-Jones was able to initiate an Out-patient Clinic once a week at Ryde Hospital, and shortly before this he had a Mental Welfare Clinic which also became a Child Guidance service at County Hall. About this time also a small laboratory came into use in the hospital, and the private patient block was converted into an admission block. Other changes at the hospital were the switch over to main electricity supply and the introduction of a refrigerator in the kitchen. Occupational centres were started in Newport and a year later in Ryde. There was an endeavour to make the wards more homely, to eliminate locked doors, and to encourage open air nursing on the verandas when the weather permitted. Entertainments for the patients were welcomed.

The Council planned to provide 100 places for mental defectives. The Superintendent's dominating interest was perhaps in the Mental Welfare Clinic. Mention is made in his report of prolonged depression and lassitude after influenza. There were serious epidemics of influenza in the 1930s, and those with long memories can easily recall the severe depression which sometimes followed the illness. Possibly this now would be called ME. A new Mental Welfare Clinic was opened at Northwood.

During this decade there was a steady increase in the proportion of temporary and voluntary patients admitted and treated. The number of patients rose to 390 and overcrowding of the hospital increased. The residents included 66 patients classified as mental defectives who were still in need of accommodation elsewhere. In 1937-38, 130 patients were admitted, 88 were discharged and 27 died (usually a large proportion of deaths were in patients over 70 years of age - about one half of them). A flat was now provided for a third Medical Officer and a nurses home, much needed, was planned; there were by now 23 male and 33 female nurses. The home was designed by the County Architect, Mr. Sydney Gregor, and accommodated 55 nurses; also a new hot water system was installed throughout the hospital. A holiday Camp at Brighstone for patients was considered to be an unqualified success. A social club for the staff was opened.

After the outbreak of war, the number of resident patients reached 400, and the recreation hall was fitted to take 40 male beds, and a sanitary annexe was constructed.

The accounts for this last year before the war may be of some interest.

| Income | | Expenditure | |
|---|---|---|---|
| County Patients | £27014 | Medical Staff | £1867 |
| Other ('Out-county' Patients) | £691 | Nursing Staff | £8776 |
| Paying Patients | £3095 | Other Staff | £4095 |
| Service Patients | £608 | Superannuation | £1453 |
| | | Drugs & Appliances | £480 |
| | | Clothing for Patients | £541 |
| | | Clothing for Staff (Uniforms) | £243 |
| | | Provisions | £7949 |
| | | Fuel, lighting, water & laundry | £5666 |
| Total | £31308 | | £31070 |

# V

## THE ROYAL NATIONAL HOSPITAL VENTNOR

The story of the R.N.H. Ventnor has already been told, and I include here a short chapter about it in order that this book may cover the whole ground indicated in its title.

The hospital was founded in 1868 and opened in 1869, - at which time the Royal Isle of Wight Infirmary at Ryde had been in action for 20 years and the House of Industry and its satellite infirmary for nearly a century; but none of the other hospitals except the military hospitals and Parkhurst Prison Hospital had as yet been built.

The founder was Arthur Hill Hassall, - a physician and naturalist of distinction, whose earlier works had included the first book on Human Histology (in which the structures known as Hassall's Corpuscles in the Thymus gland were first described), a book on the examination of urine; a long series of important papers in the *Lancet* on the contamination of water supplies in London and the adulteration of food, for which he received public recognition and accord; a very large number of papers on fresh water and salt water micro-organisms; and a two volume work on *British Fresh Water Algae*; he was a member of the Royal College of Physicians and a fellow of the Linnean Society. Illness brought him to Ventnor in 1866 and the next year he conceived the idea of founding a hospital for diseases of the chest.

The hospital was built between 1869 and 1878, Thomas Hellyer of Ryde being the Architect; there were eight separate blocks in a line east to west, each of which originally held 12 patients; they were in two groups of four with the hospital chapel of St. Luke dividing the two groups; later between 1885 and 1897 three additional and rather larger blocks were built to the west of the original eight; the first of these contained the large dining hall, the hospital kitchens on the top floor, offices and staff quarters. Later again there was in-filling between the original blocks, with the spaces filled in providing an operating theatre, an X-ray room and dark room and a number of single rooms, and forming two long buildings with sitting rooms and offices and other rooms on the ground floor and wards on the two upper floors; the total number of beds was raised to about 140. The kitchen garden and grounds and farm occupied in all about 26 acres; pigs and poultry were kept right up to 1948 and after, and

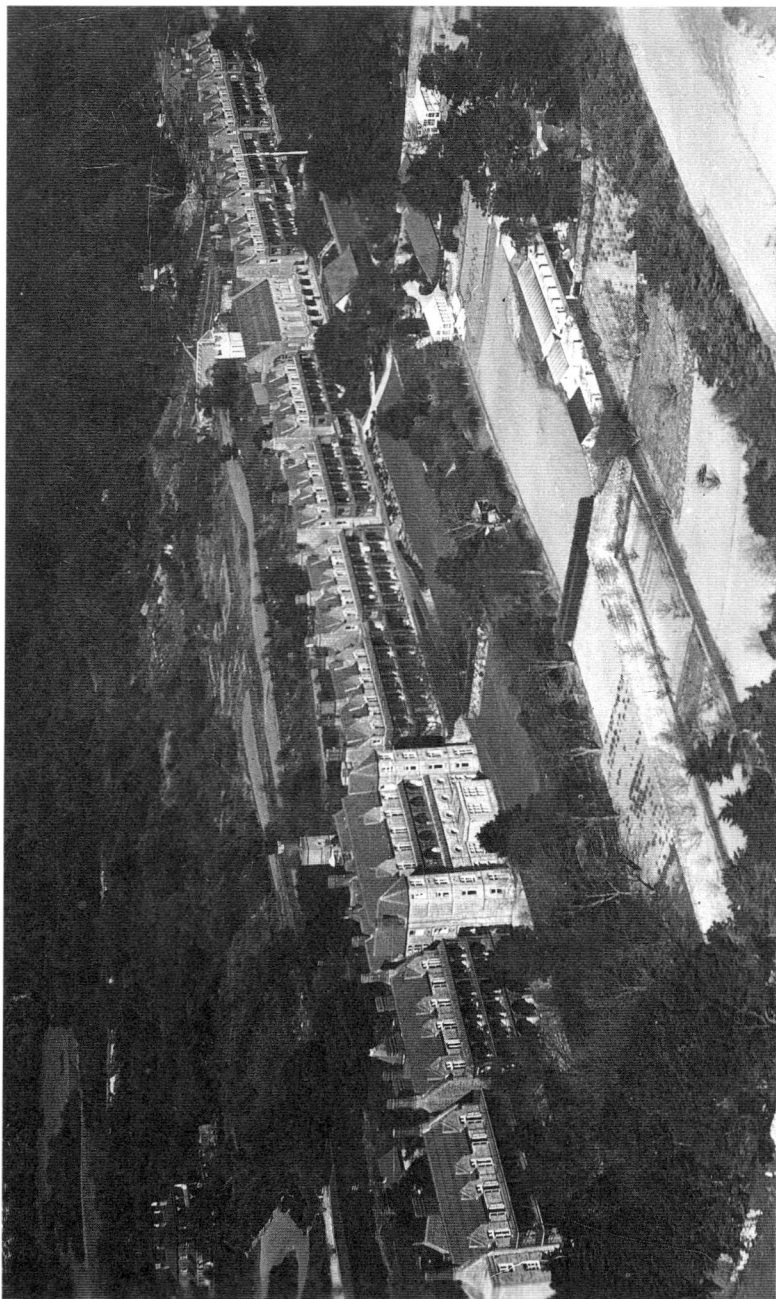

**Plate 10.** The Royal National Hospital. A panoramic view. Closed in 1964 and later demolished, the hospital and its grounds are now replaced by the Ventnor Botanic Garden. *Courtesy: R.G. McInnes.*

a good proportion of the hospital's needs in vegetables and soft fruit was grown in the grounds. In 1926 a nurses' home, the Lampard Green Home, was opened by the Prince of Wales, with accommodation for about 35 nurses, and after the war, but before 1948, a small house, Tanglewood, was bought and provided a few quiet rooms for night staff and a Matron's flat. Two houses were taken, one of them already built, for the Medical Superintendent, and one built for his Assistant within the grounds.

The Board of Management was composed mainly of professional and business men in London, and it met in the London office; there was a local or visiting committee which was authorised to deal with day to day matters; the first President was Lord Eversley - 1868 to 1882, followed by HRH Prince Leopold Duke of Albany - 1882 to 1884; the Earl of Rosebery - 1884 to 1929, and Lord Ebbisham - 1929 to 1948. The first Chairman was Sir Lawrence Peel, a retired Indian judge who lived in Bonchurch and who gave, over the years, much time and consideration to the grounds and gardens. Admission was by letter of recommendation which could be obtained from a Governor, commonly through the hospital Secretary; and by a medical certificate obtained from one of a group of doctors appointed at first chiefly in London, but within a few years widespread throughout the country.

Patients came from all regions of the country; records show that by 1938 there had been something over 38,000 patients; nearly half had come from London and Middlesex, and 14 other counties had sent more than 500; a few hundred came from Wales, Scotland and Ireland, and a number from the Channel Islands and the Continent and Dominions.

Almost all the patients were suffering from Tuberculosis, although Hassall had always intended that patients with other chest diseases should also be treated; in the early years the diagnosis was less exact and before the causative organism of Tuberculosis was known, a number of other chest complaints such as Bronchitis were treated; but it was not until after the Second World War when surgical treatment was introduced that other chest complaints were intentionally admitted for treatment.

The medical staff at the start included one resident who, like his opposite number in Ryde, also did some secretarial duties; by the turn of the century there were two or three residents, the number of patients having by now risen to 140. Hassall was from the start what we would now call the consultant physician and he attended regularly for the first few years and wrote the annual reports. Among the early residents were Dr J.M. Williamson, who after three years at the hospital went into general practice in Ventnor, where he was followed by his son; and Dr Robertson, who also practised in Ventnor for many years and who became a member of the Hospital Board and visiting physician. He was also Chairman of Longford Hospital Committee when it was first founded.

Hassall retired in 1876 and was followed by Dr J.G. Sinclair Coghill who remained as consultant and senior member of the medical staff for rather over 20 years until he died suddenly in 1899. After that no one took that position as Superintendent for the time being; the senior resident wrote the annual reports and there were local visiting physicians, in particular Dr Robertson and Dr Whitehead, the Historian of the Undercliff and one of the leading doctors on the Island; and later Dr Armstrong from Niton who with Dr Whitehead served especially through the long years of the First World War.

Meanwhile, the administration of the hospital as a whole was in the hands of a general superintendent, at first Col. Lyon Campbell, then Major Khyber Paine, and finally Mr. J.M. de Vine who retired, a sick man in 1922. After that a Medical Superintendent became the overall manager of the hospital, Dr Hutchinson; Dr Hempson in 1927; and Dr A.K. Miller in 1942.

Besides these, there were consultant physicians on the Hospital Board in London who visited the hospital professionally; there were five or six consultants and they used each to visit twice yearly so that there was a regular consultant service; many of them were on the staff at the Brompton Chest Hospital with which the R.N.H. was always glad to be loosely associated.

The National Insurance Act of 1912 led to some modification in the system of admission; patients requiring treatment for Tuberculosis now had the right to institutional treatment and every county and county borough had to provide it; arrangements for payment were reached with County Councils who thereafter paid an agreed sum for most of the patients; a small number of private patients was still admitted according to the old system, but they, if they had difficulties in paying, were provided for after a few weeks by a fund established early in the 1870s, the Hamilton Fund.

After the First World War, treatment and management evolved more rapidly than in the first 50 years of the hospital's life. Routine X-rays began in the 1920s; until the introduction of the N.H.S., all radiographic work was done by the doctors. The development of the various techniques described collectively as Collapse Therapy led to the introduction of major thoracic surgery, and visiting surgeons attended at monthly and later at fortnightly intervals for several years, until in 1940 the war brought this to a close for the time being.

Early in the Second World War, the number of beds was substantially increased by converting all but few of the rooms which up to then had all been single, to hold two patients instead of one; thereafter the hospital was able to take about 250 patients.

At the start of the war, as had been previously arranged, most of the patients were sent home, and a number of the remainder were taken to two converted holiday camps near Bembridge; this venture was not a great success, the first winter of the war was a bitterly cold one; within a few months the demand for large numbers of beds for casualties had gone into abeyance, and the hospital was soon filled again and the camps closed.

After the war, surgery was resumed in 1947, Mr. N.F. Adeney coming from Boscombe once a fortnight with his anaesthetist; Dr Miller did minor surgical operations as required. There were now three resident doctors, as well as the Superintendent and his assistant. The Management Board continued to meet in London, visiting the hospital once yearly for an annual inspection; but now members of the Local Committee were mostly elected onto the Management Board. During the short interval between the resumption of surgery and the start of the N.H.S., a beginning was made in operating upon respiratory diseases other than Tuberculosis; but at that time Tuberculosis was still by far the most important problem for anyone working in chest diseases; and it still dominated the scene; there was a painfully long waiting list; the LCC had by arrangement about 80 beds in the hospital and Middlesex County Council had 36; the other home counties usually sent a number of patients, but a few came from far and wide, including two from Spain and one from the Falkland Isles.

Physiotherapy had necessarily accompanied surgical treatment and occupational therapy which had been started during the war by voluntary workers became a regular activity. The farm and vegetable and fruit garden continue in use. The names given to the wards in the last few decades of the hospital's life commemorated the founder, Hassall, two of the Presidents, Eversley and Ebbisham, and other donors, Leaf, Hargrove, Nunn, Burgoyne and Hamilton.

The Leaf family, one or other of them, was associated with the hospital from its foundation to the day when it was taken over into the Isle of Wight Hospital Management Committee in 1958; Mrs. Hamilton gave much of the money for the building and the furnishing of the chapel and endowed the fund available to support private patients; the Hargroves were solicitors to the hospital for most of its life; Mr. F. Crompton-Nunn who followed his father as a member of the Board gave money for the building of the chapel tower and for the in-filling which joined the blocks and which provided the operating theatre and X-ray department; and the Burgoyne family were members of the Board from the start up to 1948, Treasurer and Chairman for many years, and gave the patients' library building, one of the few parts of the hospital still now in use (as a tourist shop).

(Since the hospital's life did not extend very far into the years of the N.H.S., it seems best to deal with its remaining time in this single chapter.)

When July 1948 came, the Management Board was of course replaced by the Hospital Management Committee subordinate to its regional board, at that time the South West Metropolitan Region. Little changed in the staff; the hospital constituted a group all on its own and remained for a decade separate from the other Island hospitals which were united as the I.o.W. Hospital Group; the hospital Secretary became the group secretary and the Medical Superintendent the Physician Superintendent who continued in his work, but also became Consultant Chest Physician to the Island, visiting Longford Hospital to confer with the Island Chest Physician regularly, and available to see patients in consultation with general practitioners and with other consultants when required.

The big developments which took place at the R.N.H. in the next 10 years were a result of the discovery and use of effective drugs in the treatment of Tuberculosis; they happened to take place in the first few years of the NHS, but were really entirely independent of this. The use of Streptomycin and Paramino-Salicylic acid and later of Isoniazid, by means of which tuberculous infection could be controlled and eliminated led at first to a great increase in surgical treatment; cardio-thoracic surgery was in any case developing rapidly in the early 1950s and a new thoracic surgical centre was planned at Southampton; while this was being built and the Director of Thoracic Surgery there, Mr. E.F. Chin was supervising it, he or his senior registrar worked for a time at Ventnor; and the years from 1952 to 1955 were the busiest and most active years of the whole of the hospital's life.

As the regional centre at Southampton developed, Mr. H.M. Bradmore, a member of the Regional Team who led a branch of the Thoracic Surgical Service centred at Portsmouth, took over the work at Ventnor. After a few years during which the proper management of the anti-tuberculous drugs was learned it became apparent that surgical treatment would only very seldom be needed for Tuberculosis. Meanwhile, however, other respiratory disorders were being treated at the R.N.H. to an increasing extent, although work was mainly confined to Island patients, the hospital tending towards a local function rather than a national one; a few cases from Portsmouth were brought over for surgical treatment at the R.N.H.; and a number of beds were regularly occupied by non-tuberculous patients.

By 1958 the hospital had about 100 empty beds; the demand for beds for patients with Tuberculosis having fallen very rapidly. In 1955 Longford Hospital was no longer required as a Tuberculosis sanatorium and was taken out of action and the few remaining patients there were transferred to Ventnor; and soon after that Dr Miller and his assistant at the R.N.H. took over the clinic work now carried on at St. Mary's which hitherto had been done by the Chest Physician, who was also resident and superintendent at Longford, Dr Easton; he left to take up an appointment in Glasgow and for a short time a small accessory out-patient clinic was managed as well at Ventnor.

In 1958 the Physician Superintendent was directed to leave the hospital and to work as Consultant Physician in the Island group with beds at St. Mary's and the County Hospital; his assistant was asked to carry on and manage the hospital which it was intended to close in about a year. Things did not turn out quite like that, for although the demand due to Tuberculosis was very much less than it had been, other conditions - chronic Bronchitis, Cancer of the lung, these two both so closely related to cigarette smoking, and asthma were becoming of greater significance and on a small scale more beds were needed for these. In the end the hospital carried on for about six years and was finally closed in 1964.

In 1948 the Hospital Management Committee had been made up to a great extent of those members who had previously been on the Local Committee, many of them also on the Management Committee in London, and Col. Edward Leaf the Chairman of that Committee was invited to and agreed to join the new H.M.C.. Mr. Whillier was the first Chairman and he was followed by Mr. Netherton and then by General Roome who was also Chairman then of the Isle of Wight H.M.C.. Finally in 1958 the two Management Committees were merged and after 90 years the R.N.H. ceased to have its own independent existence; and not many years after that passed into disuse, if not oblivion. It closed finally in 1964; for five years no use was found for it and both buildings and grounds became to an increasing extent a wilderness. Then the local council, happily rejecting suggestions of a housing estate or holiday camp, determined, helped perhaps by suggestions from others, to develop an open garden there. The grounds underwent a metamorphosis and with the help of Sir Harold Hillier became Ventnor Botanic Garden.

# VI

## LONGFORD HOSPITAL - HAVENSTREET

In October 1919, the County Medical Officer (C.M.O.) was asked to prepare a scheme for dealing with Tuberculosis among the Island population, - in particular for hospital treatment where it was needed for both insured and uninsured persons. (Insured persons were known at that time, and for many years to come, as panel patients). Several possible sites were considered, and in June 1920 Councillor Ball was authorised and empowered to attend a sale by auction of Longford House, and to purchase it for the Council; in September it was duly acquired for £3,000; and a month later the Council purchased the freehold of the house and grounds, including its timber, for £925.

Longford House had been the Island residence of John Rylands, a wealthy Lancastrian industrialist from Longford Hall near Manchester; in Havenstreet village he also built the Longford Institute, - later known as Holmdale - as a sort of club and library for the village; it enters briefly into this story during the Second World War; and he also built a gas works which supplied the village as well as his own house. He died in 1888.

The house needed a good deal of work before it was suitable for its purpose and had to be enlarged; an early plan to provide more beds in a wooden pavilion was rejected by the Ministry and in June 1921 it was agreed that a new block to contain 16 beds should be built to supplement the existing accommodation. Meanwhile the R.N.H. at Ventnor offered to take Island patients at three guineas per patient per week; beds were also available at this time at Hawthorndene in Bonchurch and at the Hermitage. The former later became an outpost of the LCC and accommodated about 30 convalescent girls and women, medical care being provided by the local practitioners and supervision in respect of their Tuberculosis by Dr Miller who visited weekly; the patients were brought to the R.N.H. for X-rays and occasionally admitted for treatment. The Hermitage, sometimes know as Dr Bassano's Hospital or sanatorium, was (and is) a rather remote building high up at the north end of St. Catherine's Down; Dr Bassano was a practitioner in Ventnor, who did some work in pathology at the R.N.H.. The Hermitage continued to function as a nursing home until about the end of the Second World War.

In August 1921 Dr D. Morrison-Smith was appointed Tuberculosis Officer and Assistant C.M.O. and was to be the Medical Officer at Longford Hospital; work on the building continued through 1921 and much of 1922; electric lighting was installed, but this necessitated the hospital having its own generator; and, as seems often to have been the case on the Island, the water supply caused some problems. The Matron took office in May 1922, but had to be found rooms for a time in Holmdale House. Dr Morrison-Smith wished to resign in August 1922, but agreed to stay on until the end of September; and the hospital was officially opened on August 10th 1922 by Dr Robertson of Ventnor, Chairman of its committee; the next month there were 11 patients, 8 of them women - in residence. The staff included, besides the Matron, one sister, two staff nurses or charge nurses, a cook general, two ward maids, one girl coming in daily, a laundress and a handyman.

A report had to be made to the Committee of any patient who was detained more than eight weeks. The C.M.O. reported to the Committee that 'Wherever patients are able to contribute to their maintenance they are expected to do so, and as a rule this is done willingly'. An Out-patient Clinic was held at the hospital, but in 1923 a clinic was opened at County Hall, - as it was felt (no doubt quite correctly) that patients would find it easier to attend there than at Longford, and a shed at the rear of County Hall was converted into a clinic for this and for a Venereal Disease Clinic; later that year Tuberculosis health visiting became available. Paying patients could be admitted to Longford provided accommodation was available at a charge of £2.50 per week.

The hospital was administered by the Sanatorium Sub Committee of the Public Health Committee of the County Council; Dr Robertson who first came to Ventnor as a resident at the R.N.H. about 1880 was its Chairman. In the 1930s the hospital held 45 patients and shortly before the war a further 14 beds were added when the Rev. W.E. Bowen gave in memory of his wife the Catherine Bowen Home, a new building placed within the hospital grounds but a little way from the main building.

At this stage Dr Carpenter, as Assistant C.M.O., supervised the services for Tuberculosis; his report to the Committee each month included not only the admissions, discharges and bed occupancy; the staff numbers and changes; but also the weight and market value of the vegetables grown in the hospital garden and the number of eggs laid each month by the hospital poultry.

The Tuberculosis service carried on during the war and after it until the National Health Service. As was the case with the R.N.H. this function ceased after a few years and it seems best to complete the story here. Dr Easton succeeded Dr Carpenter and lived in a house adjacent to the hospital which he superintened while he also worked as Chest Physician on the Island, holding clinics after 1948 first at County Hall and then from 1952 at St. Mary's in the new wing of the Out-patient building.

The Catherine Bowen Home was by 1954 not thought suitable for children, and by then in any case there were not many children requiring institutional treatment for Tuberculosis; it was closed for the time being and the few children needing hospital care were sent to the Whitehouse Sanatorium at Milford on the mainland. The need for hospital beds for Tuberculosis declined steadily and early in 1955 Longford Hospital ceased to be a sanatorium; the few patients left there were transferred to the Royal National Hospital in Ventnor; the Superintendent there and his assistant took on the chest clinic work and Dr Easton took up an appointment near Glasgow.

VII

## THE FRANK JAMES HOSPITAL

The story of this hospital is well known in East Cowes, Cowes and the Island generally, and an account of the tragic death of Frank James in 1890 has been given recently by Helga Foxcroft. For the information that I have about the hospital I am particularly indebted to Mrs. Elizabeth (Heather) Gray, the last Administrator of the hospital who tells me that her Great Uncle was one of the first; also to other members of the staff still serving in the hospital.

Frank Linsly James was the son of a wealthy Liverpool merchant; he kept a yacht, the *Lancashire Witch,* at Cowes; the guilded weather-vane atop the roof of the hospital is a representation of this yacht.

The Frank James Memorial Home was built in his memory by his two brothers, Arthur and William, on land given for the purpose, as a home for aged and disabled seamen and their wives and mainly composed of a series of single and double cabins; and so it remained for about six years. An inscription in stone above the entrance read:

'Ye who in these walls do meet,
Pray you find a safe retreat,
tho' ye fought with wind and tide,
here in Port may ye abide.
Till that day your voyage be,
whither is nor storm nor sea.'

Then in 1899 there was need for a convalescent home for soldiers from the South African War; the residents were given pensions and found accommodation elsewhere, and the home taken over for this purpose. After about three years this need faded out, and it was then suggested to the brothers by Princess Beatrice that it would be of value as a local hospital. The brothers offered to endow it, provided that after a trial of two years they were satisfied with the management and maintenance of the hospital; meanwhile they made an allowance of £300 a year for it.

So on June 25th 1903 the Frank James Hospital was opened by Princess Beatrice, Governor of the Island. Her signature appears in the Visitors' Book

115

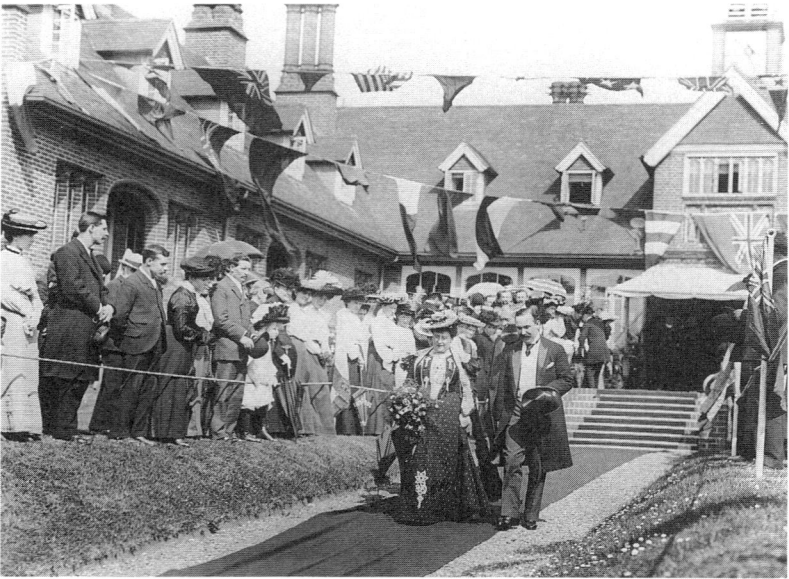

**Plate 11**. The opening of the Frank James Hospital by Princess Beatrice June 25th 1903. *Courtesy: Beken of Cowes & Mrs. E. Gray.*

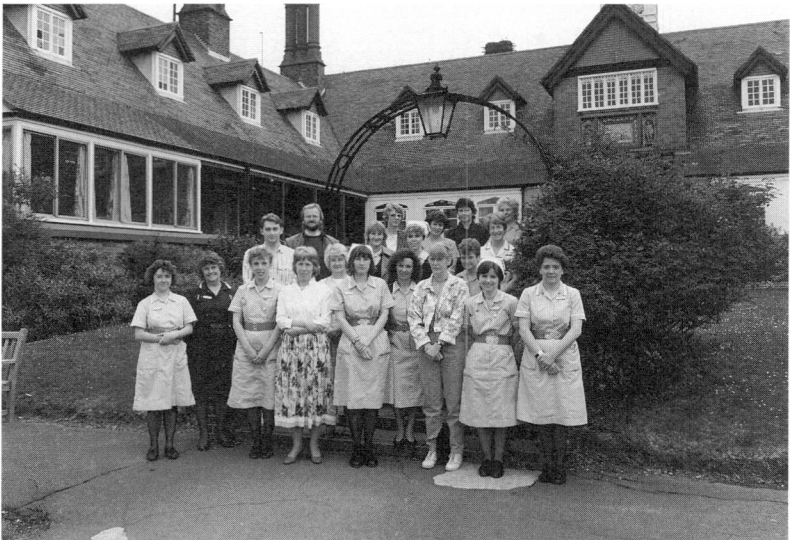

**Plate 12**. The Frank James Hospital with some of its staff. *Courtesy: Mrs. E. Gray.*

and is followed immediately by those of Arthur and William James. Regrettably this book is no longer to be seen in the hospital.

Satisfied with its performance after two years, Arthur and William James endowed it with £10,000; a trust was set up of five members including John Arthur James and E.G. Carnt Esq., and was supplemented by the sum of £766 handed over by the Trustees of the Cowes Cottage Hospital Scheme, the sum rounded up to £800 by Mr. E.G. Carnt. The land and building were handed over to the Trust on January 8th 1906. Thereafter the Frank James was very much a local hospital supported by the local population and most especially for many years, so long as it existed, by the firm and employees of J.S. White, who made very many contributions and gifts.

In 1909 they gave funds for the installation of X-ray apparatus and also furniture and fittings to make a small four bedded childrens' ward. Princess Beatrice remained President of the hospital and among many other local names those of Mr. Mundell who collected funds, and of Mr. W. Ball, the Treasurer who gave advice on structural alterations, and Mr. E.G. Carnt and his brother W.G. Carnt of Manchester Royal Infirmary who gave advice about the X-ray installation, may be mentioned.

The year's income of the hospital reported upon at the annual meeting of 1910 was £1,790-5s-7d; £300 of this was given by the employees of J.S. White for the above X-ray installation and childrens' ward, and tribute was paid to Lee Densham Esq. who opened the ground of Norris Castle to the public at the Naval review the previous year, the admission charges giving the hospital £61.

Expenditure for that year was £1,692; the cost of the X-ray installation and childrens' ward had amounted to £334-15s-3d; £200 had been put in the emergency fund; nursing salaries were £183, and other salaries amounted in all to £85-15s-7d including the gardener; dressings, drugs and appliances cost £73-12s-10d; ale and stout, wine, spirits and minerals £28-8s-5d; provisions in all £370-18s-4d; fuel and light £122-9s-7d.

154 patients had been admitted that year and 156 discharged. The average stay was just under 21 days which indicates that the bed occupancy must have been just about 11, presumably the total number of beds was somewhat more than this, - perhaps 14 or 15. 37 patients were classified as medical, 107 as surgical, and 11 as dental; 99 came in on their doctor's recommendation, 25 as a result of accidents; 18 were emergency admissions; 14 were paying patients; and 9 had Typhoid Fever. 5 patients died; 130 were discharged, cured, and 16 relieved; 5 left at their own request, and 9 remained in hospital. 96 came from Cowes, 39 from East Cowes, 19 from Whippingham, Osborne, Gurnard and Northwood, and 4 from yachts and 7 from elsewhere.

An operating theatre was provided in 1912; Dr Mayo, a practitioner in Cowes did the first operation.

In 1938 a large addition was built at the south end of the hospital providing a 12 bedded ward for men with an annexe which served, at times anyhow, as a day/smoking room. This was opened by Sir Godfrey Baring and was known as the George V Memorial Wing.

The local practitioners of East Cowes and Cowes provided the medical staff and had the right to admit and treat their patients there; they worked a rota so that one was always available on call. There was no official out-patient department, but local minor casualties would go there as an alternative to the doctor's surgery and would be dealt with, - as happened in other such local hospitals; in those days the population in the neighbourhood of a hospital always expected it to provide a service for casualties.

As the different special departments became operative at the County Hospital and elsewhere, - E.N.T., Ophthalmic, Orthopaedic, Pathology, etc., consultants dealing in these matters would visit the hospital when their advice was sought.

Right up to 1948 the hospital was dependent to a degree upon local contributions; in 1910 annual subscriptions had yielded £140; workshop collections £367, congregational collections £36, entertainments £29, in all nearly one third of the total income; paying patients had yielded £217 and interest on shares, the endowment, £343; it is not surprising that Cowes was unwilling to join in the contributory scheme which the Royal County Hospital set up in 1936, - it had its own in place. Anyone going into the Frank James now is soon aware of its association with the community, and with East Cowes most particularly.

# VIII

## THE SHANKLIN HOSPITALS

There were three small hospitals in Shanklin; the first of these to be established was the 'Scio Hospital and Surgical Home for Children', in Scio House, Atherley Road, close to the railway station. The hospital was built and endowed by Mrs. Scaramanga of Westhill in 1891 in memory of her two sons; she was a member of the Ralli family and after her death the hospital and its contents and her endowment of it passed in the form of a trust to the care of her two brothers and in due course was passed on by them to a trusteeship of three local Shanklin men and the local branch of Lloyds Bank. It was the only hospital for children on the Island and treatment was free. The Honorary Medical Staff were Dr Dabbs and Dr John Cowper who was the surgeon and the Matron was Miss Emma Durham.

In 1910 Scio House moved to Arthur's Hill. In 1940 one of the three trustees was Mr. W.T.W. Somers who had been acting as Honorary Secretary; he left some records for an incoming secretary in which he discusses the finances of the hospital and the staffing. The staff at that time consisted of the Matron, one sister, one assistant nurse, one senior probationer, and two probationers together with one cook and a gardener. He mentioned that nurses seldom stayed very long and often had to be hired from Southsea Nursing Homes at a charge of three guineas a week. The difficulty of course was that nurses in a small place like that got relatively little experience and little prospect of any promotion.

The endowment left by Mrs. Scaramanga provided an income equal to only about one third of the running costs of the hospital; the rest had to be found from donations, subscriptions, etc. The contributory scheme introduced at the County Hospital in the 1930s provided that any contributors who were admitted, or whose children were admitted, to Scio House would be paid for at the rate of 6s daily for up to ten weeks. Records of admissions and discharges were noted and sent to the County Hospital quarterly and this provided quite an important source of the hospital's income. That apart there were a number of donations though the only regular one came from Miss Damon, the Head Mistress of Upper Chine School; church and school collections, the Shanklin Carnival and collection boxes at Scio House itself and elsewhere in the town had to make up the rest. Endowment funds could not be used for capital expenditure, but there was a small amount of money available for this which was used to purchase a portable X-ray apparatus and other equipment. There were at this time ten beds in the hospital, two four bedded wards for girls and boys and two single wards for private patients. Some surgery, at least in emergency, was available and I have an acquaintance who recalls being taken in there at the age of 17 about 1927 for emergency appendicectomy.

Mr. Somers, writing early in the war, when the E.M.S. was about to take over the hospitals, anticipated that a first-aid post would be set up at Scio House and the patients transferred to the 'Home of Rest'. I am not sure whether this was done, but certainly Scio House continued to function for a short time after the war and indeed was asked to take children from the County Hospital while the childrens' ward there was being redecorated. After 1946 it became a home for nurses working in the other Shanklin Hospitals and continued this function until about 1955 when it was sold and became, and now remains, a nursing home.

Winchester House at the north end of Shanklin (the Home of Rest referred to above) was originally intended as a childrens' hospital but plans were changed before it was opened and it was given by Mrs. Mary Nunn-Harvey - a member of the family of Nunn who founded the lace factory at Newport - to Winchester Diocese as a home for the Girls Friendly Society; during the Second World War as indicated it was taken over and used for a time as an emergency hospital.

The Arthur Webster Memorial Hospital in Landguard Manor Road was presented to the town by Lord Alverstone (Richard Webster) then Lord Chief Justice, who was also Chairman of the Royal National Hospital; it was in memory of his son Arthur who had died at the age of 28 and whose widow had suggested the idea of a cottage hospital for the town as a memorial; a large contribution to it came also from the trustees of the Harriet Parr bequest, - she was a local authoress who had died in 1900. The memorial tablet composed by Dr Dabbs, the Chairman of the trustees, and at that time the Doyen of the Shanklin doctors, can still be seen in the entrance hall of the hospital. At the start, the hospital had six beds in two wards together with an operating theatre, dispensary, kitchen, dining and sitting rooms and domestic quarters. It is said that it was very soon fully occupied, which was taken to indicate and confirm the need that existed for it. The hospital was opened in 1905 by Princess Beatrice, Governor of the Island, and this was a great occasion for Shanklin. In 1930 the Shanklin Rotary Society collected funds for an extension to the hospital. When the hospital was taken over by the E.M.S. early in the Second

World War it was decided that it should no longer be used for in-patients, but it has continued since then, as a clinic, with a dental surgery and especially a centre for physiotherapy, an outpost for the pathological laboratory services, and an ambulance garage.

The third hospital in Shanklin was opened as a private convalescent home, Maycroft, in 1925 by Lilian Lainsbury; the house had formerly belonged to Mr. J. Charles Wadham. It was in use then and through the Second World War as a private nursing home, but in 1946 it was purchased and taken over by the board which was then in control of the Arthur Webster Hospital and Scio House; it then became the Shanklin Cottage Hospital. Patients were admitted by the Shanklin doctors who provided the medical care there and Mr. Gaynor was the surgeon. In 1948 of course it was taken over by the National Health Service.

# IX

## ISLE OF WIGHT ISOLATION HOSPITALS

The Notification of Infectious Diseases Act was passed in 1889 and in 1893 the Isolation Hospital Act. Both hospitals and local authorities had for a long time recognised the need for wards or separate institutions for infectious diseases and these had been provided both at Newport Infirmary and Ryde Hospital and a separate nursing staff had been appointed for these wards.

Now in 1893 the County Council recommended the local authority districts to form hospital committees and to set up isolation hospitals. Three such hospitals were established in the course of the next decade. The largest and the one with the longest life was that at Ventnor where the records are more complete than elsewhere so I mention this first.

*————— Ventnor and the Undercliff Isolation Hospital —————*

The Committee was constituted and termed 'The Undercliff Hospital Committee' by order of the County Council in 1896, holding its first meeting in the council chamber of the Ventnor U.D.C. on August 12th of that year. Among the committee members were Mr. G.F. Ingram who was elected Chairman and Major T. Khyber-Paine, the General Superintendent of the Royal National Hospital. The hospital was intended to serve Ventnor and the villages of, or close to, the Undercliff, - Bonchurch, St. Lawrence, Niton, Whitwell, Wroxall, and Godshill. The Committee decided as a temporary measure in the first place to take a house, Rookwood, in Gills Cliff Road, and work was in hand fitting this for the purpose and furnishing it; however at this stage the Hamborough Estate in which the house was located indicated unwillingness for the matter to proceed and agreed to compensate the Committee for work already done. There was some delay and searching after this, but eventually two acres of land in Upper Ventnor were leased from Captain Lowther for 999 years. Tenders were invited for the building, and no less than 81 applications were received, only 18 of them having included the deposit required; a loan of £2,320 was obtained, and later additional loans of £700, £150 and £400 were needed. It was not until 1904 that the hospital was finally opened and Mr. and Mrs. Cameron were installed as caretaker and nurse with accommodation, heating, lighting and a joint salary of 20s weekly + 5s for payment of assistants. While the hospital was being built some cases of Scarlet Fever had by agreement been sent to the Sandown and Shanklin Joint Hospital which the Committee had been to inspect before making their final plans for their own hospital. The Ventnor Hospital, properly known as the Ventnor and Undercliff Isolation Hospital, included four wards each of more than 350 square feet, together with a nurses' room, two bathrooms and two earth closets; there was also an administrative block with kitchen, a multi-purpose sitting-waiting-board room, and the mortuary block with a wash house, laundry, ambulance shed, cold store and sterilising tank, etc.; and there were living quarters for the staff. (See Fig. 8)

It was agreed from the start that cases of Smallpox should not be admitted; nevertheless in March 1905 there was an emergency over a patient who had just arrived from America with Smallpox; she had contracted the illness on board ship from another passenger; it was decided that she must be admitted despite previous decisions and her family were also admitted and isolated; they, or their representative, were asked to defray any expense if as a consequence other patients had to be sent to some other hospital.

The next year the Committee learned that it would be held responsible for damages if any patient were discharged prematurely and as a consequence the disease was spread to other people (this opinion was based upon a legal action in Liverpool). At this time and apparently for many years after, the Chairman of the Committee who, except for one year, was a layman had absolute right to admit and discharge patients from the hospital.

Inevitably admissions to the hospital were sporadic and quite irregular and the Chairman was authorised to appoint additional nurses at his discretion. After a few years the hospital, which seemed to be filling a gap in the services needed for the Island, agreed to take patients from all parts of the Island and incidentally to disinfect items sent from Ryde. Some years later in 1912 the County Council in response to an inquiry said that they had no arrangements for the isolation of Smallpox cases; it was thought that if necessary such cases could probably go to the hospital ship in Cowes.

In 1913 the Isle of Wight Joint Hospital Board inquired about the use of the Undercliff Hospital for other purposes. I believe this may have been related to the recent opening of Fairlee Hospital which came to provide all the accommodation needed for infectious diseases on the Island; and it was the case that the use of the Undercliff Hospital was slight, especially in later years. In that same year, 1913, however there was some difference in opinion between the Committee and the County Medical Officer; it seems that the C.M.O. acted without the authority of his committee in concerning himself with the functioning of the hospital; indeed it was alleged that he visited the school at Ventnor and quizzed the undertaker's seven year old little boy about the nursing at the hospital! The Camerons had stayed only for a year and their place had been taken in 1905 by Mr. and Mrs. Kemp. Mr. Kemp, the Caretaker left in 1915 joining the Army, but the hospital carried on and in 1916 was thanked by the Sandown/Shanklin Joint Hospital Board for its offer to take their patients until they had been able to appoint a new matron; however this had been done so the need did not arise.

In 1919 a telephone was installed in the hospital. It was suggested at first that it might simply have an extension of the line to the nearby cemetery.

In 1921 the Committee rejected a suggestion that the Isolation Hospital should be amalgamated with others saying that it would be pointless since the Undercliff Hospital had always been able to accommodate all the patients who needed care, and they declined an invitation to a conference on the subject - all this despite the fact that in March 1919 it was reported that no Ventnor patient had been admitted since February 1918 and only one patient from the Rural District Council in the past four or five months. Mr. Kemp died in 1922 and his wife carried on with the help of a male assistant.

In 1925 the Committee was informed that the County Council was negotiating the purchase of Osborne Isolation Hospital (this is the only reference to such a hospital that I have encountered, and I believe it may refer to the Isolation Hospital which was part of the Royal Naval College at Osborne which had been disused). The final meeting of the Committee was held in March 1935; after that the County Council took over the care and management of the hospital, but it remained in action until 1942; in fact in this last year no less than 52 patients were admitted, but there was only one diagnosis, - the Itch. There is however yet a bit more to be said about the hospital in the early days of the Health Service. It was recorded in 1939 that the hospital was served by a horse-drawn ambulance, the last one on the Island; one wonders if it was the last one in the country.

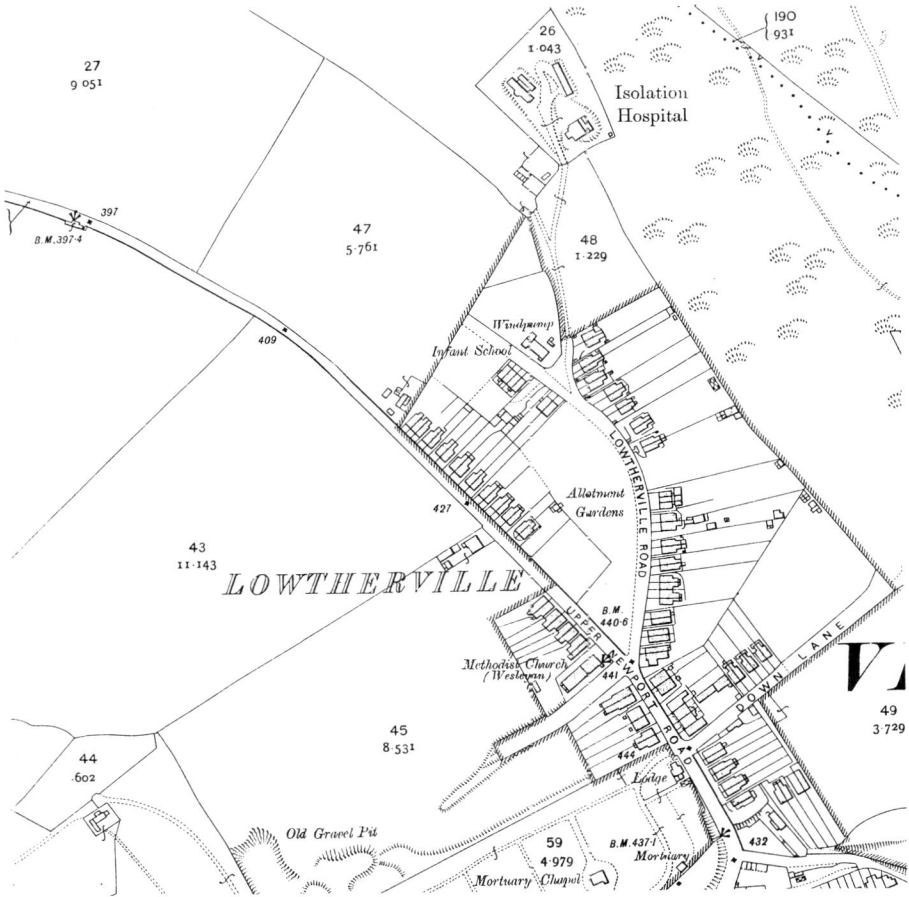

**Figure 8**. Showing the site of the Ventnor and Undercliff Hospital in Upper Ventnor. *Courtesy: Ordnance Survey.*

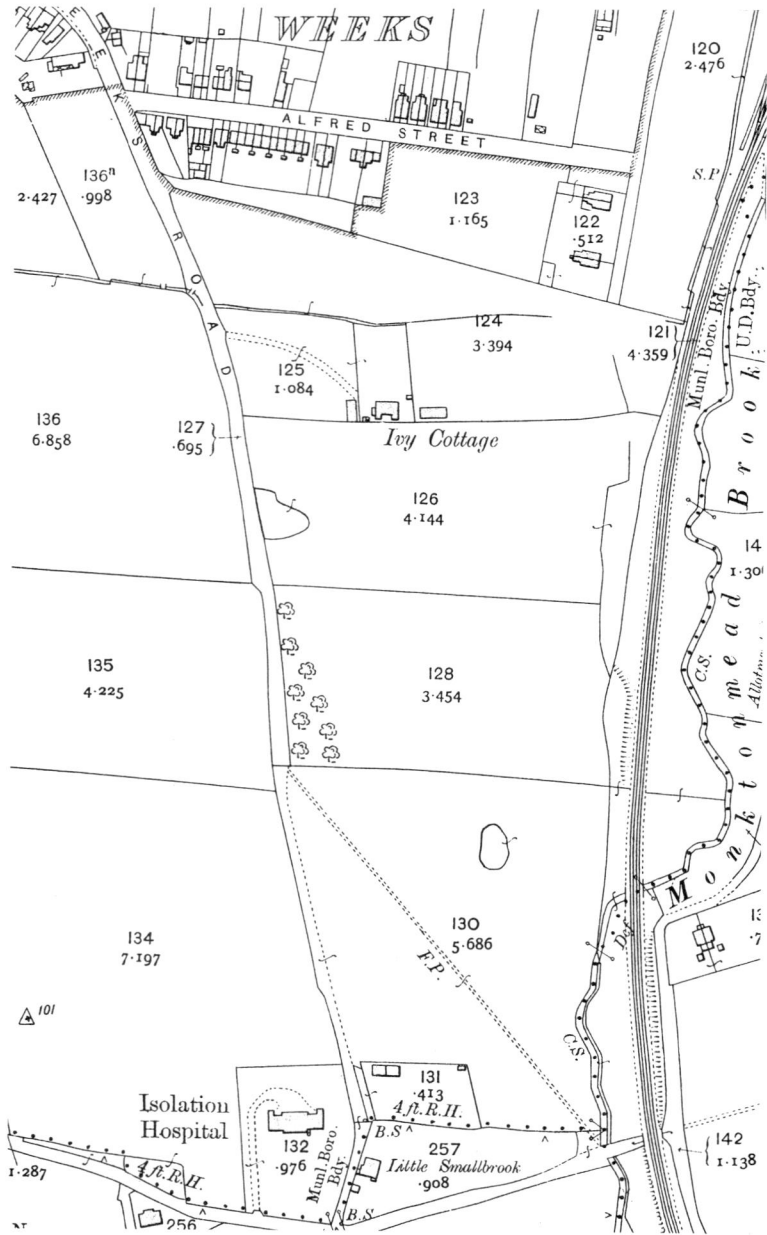

**Figure 9.** The Ryde Isolation Hospital, off Rosemary Lane.
*Courtesy: Ordnance Survey.*

So early as 1875 at a meeting of the Ryde Town Council the medical Officer of Health for Ryde reported that the Borough Hospital was in proper order for the reception of Smallpox or other infectious diseases, and that it had been empty for the past 12 months. It seems therefore that there must have been some hospital for such purposes in Ryde at that stage, - other than the Royal County Infirmary. In 1879 there is again reference to a Borough Hospital when the Medical Officer of Health, Dr A. Platts Wilkes, reported that the borough hospital would deal with infected bedding and clothing, having special apparatus for that purpose. He mentioned in this report that the birth rate and death rate in Ryde were 22 per 1,000 and 16 per 1,000, contrasting with the rates for the U.K. of 34 and 21. Infant mortality at that time in Ryde was 153 for 1,000 births. He also advised that all cases of Scarlet Fever, Smallpox, Measles, Typhus, etc. should be removed without delay to the borough hospital or the Royal Infirmary.

This hospital was a wooden structure, painted white, in the area of Ryde known as Weeks; it was known as the Small-pox hospital but was evidently available for other infections. It was moved in 1805 when Ryde Borough Council purchased land for an Isolation Hospital - about one acre off Rosemary Lane, - leased from the Manor of Ryde and Ashey, and there was set up on a brick foundation. (See Fig. 9)

An additional strip of land was leased in 1911. The hospital came to have two buildings, the wooden one with two four-bedded wards and later a brick building for an ambulance and for disinfection equipment. Some years after this hospital came into use, a letter was received from St. Helen's Urban District Council, referring to a proposal from that council and the Isle of Wight R.D.C. and the County Council, that Ryde should join them in a scheme for a new isolation hospital. Ryde responded that they already had an isolation hospital, but would be prepared to extend it to provide an additional six beds for patients from St. Helen's, but that they did not wish to join any other scheme; however this plan was found to involve too heavy a charge on the rates and was turned down.

The purchase of more land in 1911 suggests that the hospital continued for some time after this. Moreover, the records of the I.o.W. Joint Hospital Board show that it was only in 1934 that Ryde Borough was represented on that board and made a contribution to its income: it seems therefore that the Ryde Isolation Hospital may have functioned until that year. This isolation hospital was of course quite distinct from the Ashey Smallpox Hospital. (See Fig. 9)

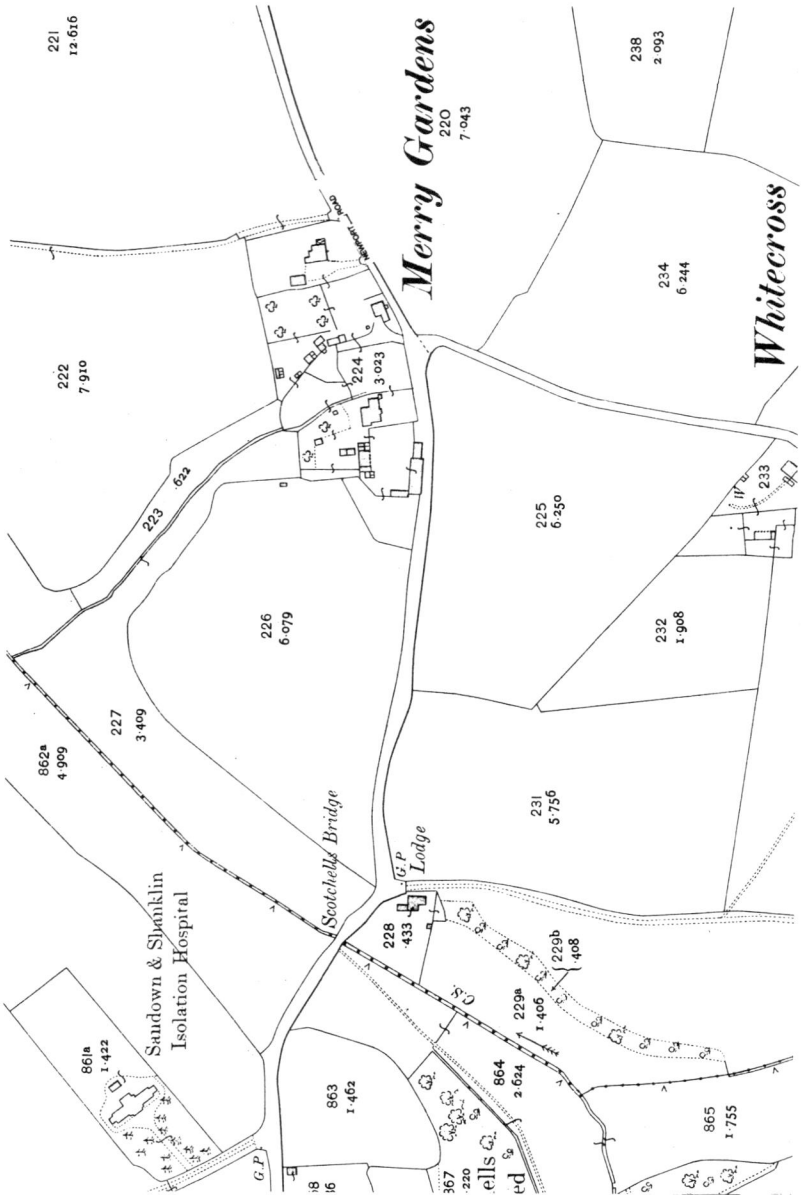

**Figure 10**. The Sandown-Shanklin Isolation Hospital, close to Scotchell's Brook. *Courtesy: Ordnance Survey.*

## The Sandown and Shanklin Joint Isolation Hospital at Scotchell's Brook

Much of the information that I have been able to collect about this hospital, which seems to have faded from memory almost entirely, - as well as about the other three Shanklin hospitals - is derived from two short books by Alan Parker, - *Victorian Shanklin* and *Shanklin Between the Wars*. So early as 1882 a joint isolation hospital for Shanklin, Sandown and Ventnor had been mooted, but got no further, until after the Isolation Hospital Act of 1893; after this Ventnor dropped out of any agreement, but Sandown and Shanklin after considerable discussion agreed upon a site of about three acres purchased from Mr. Alexander close to Scotchell's Bridge and in 1899 a hospital providing about 16 beds was built lying just on the north side of the road about 100 yards west of Scotchell's Bridge. (See Fig. 10)

Very little other information seems available about the hospital. It was enlarged in 1911, it was managed by a joint board from Sandown and Shanklin Councils and it was presumably staffed by the local doctors. In 1924 Shanklin U.D.C. wished to retain the hospital, while Sandown favoured closing it. Shanklin also incidentally recommended an isolation ward at the Arthur Webster Hospital at this time.

From 1926 to 1933 it carried on as a Shanklin concern only. The Matron, Miss F. Evans had a salary of £200 a year and the Medical Officer at this time Dr C.R. Handfield-Jones had £20 per year + 7s-6d for each visit. There was a charge of three guineas weekly for the patients. However the hospital closed in 1933, but it was on the market for several years before it was disposed of.

## Fairlee Hospital

The last and largest of the Isolation Hospitals was built a decade or so after the small ones serving the separate councils. It was created and administered by the Isle of Wight Joint Hospital Board, chaired at first by Mr. D. Dabell; unfortunately I have been unable to find the records of this Board and almost the only information about the early history of the hospital has to come from the *County Press*.

There was debate about such a hospital in Newport as early as 1902 and consideration was given to a site in Carisbrooke and later to land adjacent to Staplers Road. However eventually land from the Wickham Martin Estate was taken and Mr. J. Meader Junior of Cowes undertook to complete the building

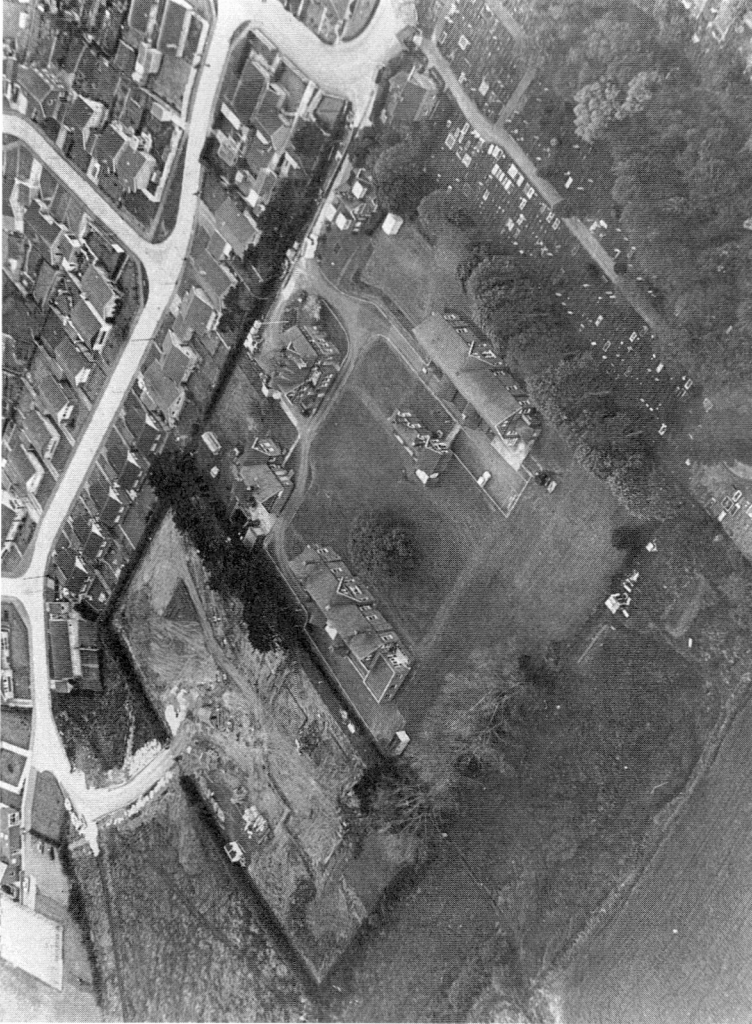

**Plate 13.** An aerial view of Fairlee Hospital - now the Mountbatten Hospice.
The small centre block was later demolished and the main block on the right has been greatly modified and extended, linking up with the lodge, and now constitutes the hospice.
Halberry Lodge has been built on the north side. *Courtesy: Pam Osborne (& others?).*

in nine months for £5,960. Arthur Gill of Newport supplied the water mains and the Isle of Wight Electric Light Company and the Newport Gas Company were responsible for the other services.

There were three main buildings, the two ward blocks each with a double ward of about 10 beds to each half; and an administrative block with kitchen, offices and living quarters for the Matron and others; these three were set on three sides of the wide lawn and at some stage a small additional block containing three separate rooms and a service room was erected in front of the western block at the edge of the lawn; it lay a few yards away from the main entrance to the western block and was serviced from there.

Besides these three buildings there was a block containing boiler house, stores and mortuary, etc. and a lodge occupied by a lodge keeper and having at the back rooms and facilities for the disinfection of clothes, etc. and public baths.

The hospital was opened in 1912. Patients were under the care of the County Medical Officer and his staff. Many changes of function and alterations of buildings were to come at Fairlee, but most of them belonged to the later part of its history in the days of the National Health Service.

However it is perhaps worth giving here a summary of Dr Fairley's list of notifications of infectious diseases for one year, that is 1935. In this year there was no Smallpox, Cerebral Spinal Fever, Poliomyelitis or Encephalitis lethargica. Scarlet Fever had the highest number of notifications, 171; others were Diphtheria - 29, Enteric Fever - 4, Pneumonia - 16, Puerperal Fever - 4, Puerperal Pyrexia - 14, Erysipelas - 28, and Ophthalmia Neonatorum - 5. There were also 66 cases of Pulmonary Tuberculosis and 27 cases of other Tuberculosis notified that year, though these of course would not have gone to Fairlee.

―――――――― *The Smallpox Hospital at Ashey* ――――――――

The isolation of patients suffering from Smallpox presented a problem for the hospitals or local authorities which had to provide it. I have been unable to find precise details of how the disused school at Ashey was taken over for this purpose in 1919, but one assumes it was by the authority of the County Council on the advice of the then C.M.O., Dr Walker.

There was an outbreak of Smallpox in Cowes and Newport in 1919. A child came to Cowes from Southampton after being discharged from the infectious diseases hospital there where she had been treated for Scarlet Fever, but had been in contact with a woman thought to have chicken pox; arrived in Cowes the child became ill and was found to have Smallpox. Twelve cases resulted in all; eight in Cowes and four in Newport; all were considered to be contacts of the child, the index case.

The presence of these cases in the Old School at Ashey caused concern to the Ryde Council; adjacent to the school was a farm which supplied milk to part of Ryde; on the advice of the Vet to the Ryde Council the farmer was required to stop supplying his milk, and the Council protested to the County Council and to the Ministry of Health, and suggested that either the Government should be asked to provide a hospital ship or alternatively a more out of the way spot somewhere on the Island. The Isle of Wight Joint Hospital Board also thought that the building at Ashey was unsuitable and inadequate and suggested that a hospital should be set up using an old army hut, which would be available, somewhere within two miles of Fairlee Hospital, which could be administered by the staff of Fairlee.

The Ministry of Health had a report upon the outbreak by the Inspector, Dr McEwen, and the Borough and County Councils asked for a copy of this report; but received the answer that the report was for the Ministry only and would not be promulgated. There was much dissatisfaction at this. The request was repeated and again refused and the Council then said they would seek to have a question asked in the House of Commons by the Isle of Wight M.P. It transpired however that he was ill and unable to attend the House at the time, but after a while another M.P. kindly took up the matter, and a question was put to the Minister of Health, Dr Addison, in Lloyd George's government, by Sir Clement Kinmont-Cook, only to receive the same answer, that the report was for the Ministry only.

There was further debate between the councils as to which of them was responsible for the expenses which had been incurred in the care of the patients treated at Ashey; the County Council seeking to divert the costs to the Borough Councils of Cowes and Newport whence the patients had come, and the Borough Councils of course maintaining that the County Council had had the obligation to provide and pay for the service. In the end the County Council had to pay the greater part of it, but the Borough Councils each had to make a contribution.

The County Council maintained throughout this dispute that the provision at Ashey was adequate and suitable and suggested that, if any of the other councils were dissatisfied with it, they should provide accommodation themselves. In the end as is well-known the hospital remained at Ashey. A deputation from the County Council visited it in 1920 and arranged for some alterations and modifications.

In 1930 a visitor to Sandown, who had been exposed to a known case of Smallpox in Enfield, before coming to the Island, became ill with a rash. He was seen by the C.M.O., Dr Fairley and his assistant, Dr Carpenter, and they also asked Dr Fraser, Medical Officer of Health of Portsmouth to come and see him here; the diagnosis of Smallpox was agreed and he was taken into Ashey Hospital on 10th April 1930. His illness was mild and he was discharged on 3rd May. The occasion was taken to overhaul and repair a number of tents and a marquee which had been stored at the hospital since 1919.

Ashey remained the Smallpox Hospital for the Island until with the elimination of the disease in the 1970s it was no long needed. It was inspected, redecorated and upgraded from time to time and electric light was provided, but so far as I know it was never in use again.

──────────── *Public Health Before, During and After* ────────────
*World War Two*

In his report for 1936, Dr Fairley, the C.M.O. gave a table showing the various Island hospitals, their function, management, number of beds available medical and nursing staff, and annual turnover of patients; a modified version of this table is shown here, giving a summary of the services available a few years before the war, and a decade or so before the N.H.S. (Table 1).

Ryde was the principle General Hospital and except for Whitecroft and the R.N.H. the only one with a resident doctor; soon after this date a second resident was appointed. The Frank James Hospital and the Arthur Webster Hospital provided beds for the local population; patients were admitted and discharged by their own practitioners, who worked a rota of on-call duties; consultants from Ryde County Hospital would see patients on request.

Scio House was a childrens' hospital with about ten beds; operative treatment was undertaken there.

The Isolation hospitals were available for infectious diseases, - Fairlee, and the Ventnor and Undercliff Hospital; Scarlet Fever, Diphtheria, Enteric Fever, and Erysipelas had been treated there during the year and Cerebral Spinal Fever and Poliomyelitis were among the notifiable diseases which would have been treated, but had not occurred that year.

Longford was the Island sanatorium for Pulmonary Tuberculosis and its beds there would soon be increased by the gift from the Rev. W.E. Bowen of the Catherine Bowen Childrens' Home. Ashey Smallpox Hospital is not mentioned in this table, but it was there, and remained available until about 1975.

Whitecroft Mental Hospital dealt with mental disorders, - there is no mention in this table of the beds at the House of Industry for mental defective patients, although they were under medical supervision both by the medical staff at St. Mary's and the psychiatrist at Whitecroft and they did have a nursing staff. The R.N.H. was, as its title says, a national hospital; it usually at this stage had a handful of patients from the Island.

The C.M.O. had two assistants (or deputies) Dr W.S. Wallace, and Dr H. Carpenter, - who concerned himself particularly with the Tuberculosis service; and two dental surgeons, Mr. L. Cartwright and Miss Hedsall. These doctors were not directly concerned with the care of patients in St. Mary's, but reference is made to the close and friendly relations between the Public Health Doctors and the hospital medical staff.

The laboratory at Ryde remained the only pathology department available on the Island and its load was steadily increasing; in 1939 they asked for financial help, but in January 1940 the Committee declined to give this, - the C.M.O. was deputed to explain the position to Mr. Aubrey-Wickham (Chairman of the RIoWCH); this refusal was confirmed and repeated three months later.

The ambulance service was provided by the Council; in 1938 there were 7 motor ambulances on the Island and at the small Ventnor isolation hospital a horse-drawn ambulance was still there. Two years later after the outbreak of war 44 ambulances were available on the Island; 6 of these were Red Cross ambulances and 11 were trade vehicles fitted out for ambulance duties.

In the years before the war there were 44 midwives in practice on the Island; 28 were employed by the District Nursing Association, 16 were independent, - 10 of them working in nursing homes; district nurses undertook ante-natal supervision in 686 cases; independent midwives paid 1,685 visits to 325 patients; Dr Linford, who joined the C.M.O.'s staff, held ante-natal clinics in Newport, Cowes, East Cowes, Freshwater and Lake; Ryde made its own arrangements.

Besides the hospital Out-patient clinics at Ryde, several clinics were held in County Hall, - for Tuberculosis (follow-up clinics); mental welfare and child guidance (also in Ryde and Northwood), and Venereal Diseases, and in 1939 a clinic for birth control was opened at County Hall apparently in response to a suggestion from Portsmouth.

There were 31 registered nursing homes on the Island, 9 of these took only maternity cases, and another 13 took maternity cases as well as others; at St. Mary's Hospital 128 maternity cases were dealt with that year.

In the committee records there is mention of such things as air-raid precautions and black-out curtains and the provision of extra beds many months before war broke out. The Emergency Medical Service (E.M.S.) took over beds in all the Island hospitals save for Longford and the Arthur Webster Hospital early in 1940. At St. Mary's beds had to be found by discharging as many patients as possible home, or transferring them to the H.o.I., - residents there being sent home; most, almost all, of the patients were aged and infirm, often very infirm; some never recovered from the move, and there was inevitable criticism and complaint in some cases. 52 patients were sent from St. Mary's to Forest House, 30 were sent home from St. Mary's, and 8 were sent home from Forest House. The initial plan was to use St. Mary's for patients from Portsmouth who needed hospital care, making beds in the large town available in case of large numbers of casualties; some 65 patients were moved from Portsmouth to the Island, 27 of them in the first two days of September 1939! It must have been a hectic time. There were 19 women and 7 infants; a few men came from East Cowes. At the same time, the Holmdale Institute in Havenstreet was taken over as an emergency maternity hospital for Portsmouth with 30 beds; this venture started on September 6th 1939 and was soon considered supererogatory and it closed on November 21st 1939; however in those eleven weeks 28 patients had been admitted and presumably about 56 discharged.

In May 1941 many windows in St. Mary's were shattered by a bomb but there were no injuries to patients or staff; and a year later came the heavy raid on Cowes, - it may have been this that led to the provision of air-raid shelters and strengthening of the 'vaults', presumably the basement at the east end of Forest House. In April 1943 another raid led to the admission of 23 patients; 4 of them died; by this time the theatre was available and surgery was provided for 10 patients.

In November 1943 the E.M.S. was requiring an allocation of 71 beds; these had to be on the ground floor there being no lift; however it seems that 38 of the 71 had been taken for ordinary patients. It was recommended that Shanklin Home of Rest (Winchester House) should be required to provide 10 beds. The next year there was a request to take surgical cases from Ryde whenever possible, to reduce the waiting list there, which might be so long as two to four months; about the same time there was mention of the need for a stock of Penicillin on the Island, - this was provided at Ryde by January 1945.

Dr Sylvester had been ill for a time during 1944 and Dr Peskett was unable single handed to cover all the necessary ground; Major Davis, R.A.M.C., from Parkhurst Barracks came and stood in for Dr Sylvester without formality, - one hopes that he and the Army received the thanks due.

After the war there was a serious shortage of nursing staff, which led to an advertisement for the appointment of ward orderlies in place of assistant nurses. The establishment recommended by the Classification Sub Committee of the P.A.C. in 1947 was for each ward of 49 beds, 1 sister, 3 staff nurses and 12 orderlies; there were also the superintendent, her deputy, and 5 relief staff; the 'surgical ward', Bonchurch, was closed. The maternity department with 11 beds and 12 cots had 1 sister, 4 midwives and 4 assistant nurses. The domestic staff for the hospital included 8 ward maids and 7 cleaners. In the wards for mental defectives, by now housing 101 patients, there were in all 4 charge nurses and 16 nursing assistants, 6 of them night workers. The Forest House at this stage held 102 men, 90 women and 26 infants in 2 nurseries; for the nurseries there were 12 foster mothers of various grades; and for the rest in all 17 orderlies, 5 of them working at night. In addition the House employed 1 stores-man; 1 dress-maker; 4 gate porters; 1 ambulance driver and 1 tailor; a laundry man and a laundry woman; 3 cooks in the main kitchen and 3 in the staff kitchen; 5 maids; 9 cleaners and 1 bath attendant. There were 13 maintenance staff, a head gardener-cum-bailiff, a second gardener and a garden labourer. Finally there was still a visiting organist whose salary was £26 per annum.

In 1946, Dr Carpenter, one of the Medical Officers of Health, died and a lady doctor, Dr Jennings, who for five years during the war had worked unpaid in the Maternity Service, retired. Dr Fairley indicated his intention of retiring and in due course Dr Wallace took his place. In a survey of the hospital services on the Island Dr Fairley said:

'There is urgent need for more beds for acute sick and maternity cases if an adequate hospital service is to be provided. The ultimate solution seems to be to build a new district hospital at Newport, - the County Hospital on a smaller scale becoming a linked local hospital. With this in view any immediate development should take place at St. Mary's Hospital, and might take the form of 150 acute beds and about 20 additional maternity beds, together with out-patient facilities, - the present premises being used for chronic sick. This would form the nucleus for a useful district hospital, as and when the County Hospital needed replacement'.

In June of the same year the Ryde Committee mentioned that the Ministry of Health had recommended various measures for the hospital, but considered that it could not expand and was not well placed for a general hospital; not surprisingly the Medical Committee disagreed.

In the County Medical Officer's report for 1949, referring to the take-over, Dr Wallace commented:

'Although when 5th July dawned, no great change became apparent in the work of my department, it would be wrong to say that no administrative difficulties were experienced. Indeed for the first few weeks, the Health Department [of County Hall] seemed to become a clearing house for the Health Executive Council and the Regional Hospital Board inquiries... Many problems remained to be solved ... The new services provided under the Act are popular, - some staggeringly so, and the demands made for example on the ambulance and home help services have caused some embarrassment, and estimates of expenditure have been made to look foolish'.

The demands on the ambulance service were all met, although there was an unexpectedly heavy demand for ambulance transport to and from the mainland which was both time consuming and expensive. In 1950 the C.M.O. regretted the transfer of responsibility for administration of the infectious diseases hospital from the Local Authority to the Hospital Management Committee. He also remarked that the major difficulty was in obtaining admission for the aged sick and subsequently discharging them. He paid tribute a year later to the good relations between the Health Department of the County Council, the hospital consultants, the General Practitioners, and the administrative officers of all departments.

Among the serious infectious diseases at that time, which did not respond to antibiotics, was Poliomyelitis; there was an epidemic in 1947 in which 46 patients were afflicted; this like the later one, was not by any means confined to the Island, - the incidence was high all over the country; in 1948 and 1949 there were relatively few cases, 7 and 9 respectively; then in 1950 came the epidemic which did so much harm to the Island, - at least for that year, and which led the media, always avid for a sensational headline, to dub the Island 'The Polio Island'; there were that year 54 cases with some paralysis and 41 non-paralytic cases notified in addition. 11 of these cases were known to have originated on the mainland; and 18 mainland cases were considered to have originated on the Island. 3 patients died and 7 in all had sufficiently severe paralysis to call for orthopaedic care. At the height of the epidemic the C.M.O. considered it wise to advise that children and young adults should not visit the Island; he mentioned, as was well known, that for every case notified and suffering from paralysis there were probably about 5 cases unnotified; in the absence of paralysis the infection produces no very characteristic symptoms; once patients have been paralysed any febrile illness with malaise may well be attributed to this infection.

## Table 1 - Hospital Services available on the Island (c.1936)

| HOSPITAL | FUNCTION | BEDS | ADMISSIONS | MANAGEMENT | MEDICAL STAFF | NURSING STAFF |
|---|---|---|---|---|---|---|
| Royal County Hospital | General | 72 | 1121 | Voluntary | 1 Resident Hon. Staff | Matron 7 staff nurses 25 Probationers |
| Frank James | General | 23 | 282 | Voluntary | Visiting | Matron - 2 Sisters 4 nurses |
| Arthur Webster | Cottage Hospital | 9 | 110 | Voluntary | Visiting | Matron 4 nurses |
| Scio House & Surgical Home | Children | 10 | 178 | Voluntary | Visiting | Matron 3 nurses |
| Royal National Hospital Ventnor | Tuberculosis | 157 | 314 | Voluntary | 3 Residents + Visiting Staff | Matron - 10 Sisters 25 nurses |
| Saint Mary's | Chronic Diseases | 128 | 184 | County Council | Visiting M.O. | 1 Sister. 2 Charge Nurses 15 Assistant Nurses |
| Saint Mary's | Maternity | 9 | 47 | County Council | Visiting M.O. | |
| Whitecroft Hospital | Mental Illness | 339 | 158 | County Council | 3 Residents + Visiting Staff | Matron 69 nurses |
| Longford Hospital | Tuberculosis | 28 | 63 | County Council | Visiting M.O. | Matron - 4 nurses |
| Fairlee Hospital | Infectious Diseases | 31 | 51 | Joint Hospital Board | Visiting M.O. | Matron - 1 Sister 4 nurses |
| Ventnor & Undercliff Hospital | Infectious Diseases | 8 | 25 | Ventnor U.D.C. | Private G.P.s | 1 + help |

X

# THE MILITARY AND NAVAL HOSPITALS

Two small military hospitals were, for a time at least, well known on the Island; and the one at Albany Barracks certainly played some part in the general life of the Island.

The barracks were built during the time of the Napoleonic wars, - around 1790 A.D. William B. Cooke in *A New Picture of the Isle of Wight* in 1808 wrote 'Not far from the House of Industry stands the barracks ..... Near it is the hospital containing a number of convenient wards, and nothing is wanting for the recovery and comfort of its afflicted inhabitants'.

The Ordnance Survey Map of 1862 (Fig 11) shows a building about 90ft x 40ft, and that of 1940 shows the same building but with additional wings on either side, and some smaller associated buildings; these occupied ground to the south-west of the main barracks and parade ground, which is now covered by a complex of roads and houses on the north side of the Forest Road; the military cemetery lies on the opposite side of the road, but in the early days there was also a small burial ground to the north-west close to the forest; what is not shown on the map is the nearby spot 'with an erected gallows, the common place of execution' which Cooke mentions.

The hospital would presumably have served whatever component of the Army was occupying the barracks at the time and possibly patients from other barracks on the Island; there were a number of occasions over the years in which its history relates to that of the Island hospitals; before St. Mary's became a hospital with facilities for surgery, the surgeons at the Albany Barracks were called in to Parkhurst Prison Hospital when operative treatment was required for patients there. Later towards the end of the Second World War when the two part-time Medical Officers to the Infirmary were in difficulties, Major Davies, as already mentioned, lent a hand and provided what medical care was needed at St. Mary's. Certainly also, after the heavy air-raid on Cowes in June 1942, a number of casualties were taken to the military hospital and treated there; and years later when orthopaedic beds were in short supply and waiting lists were lengthening, the Regional Board arranged with the authorities for a few beds to be available at the barracks hospital. The Albany Barracks were abandoned some time in the 1960s and

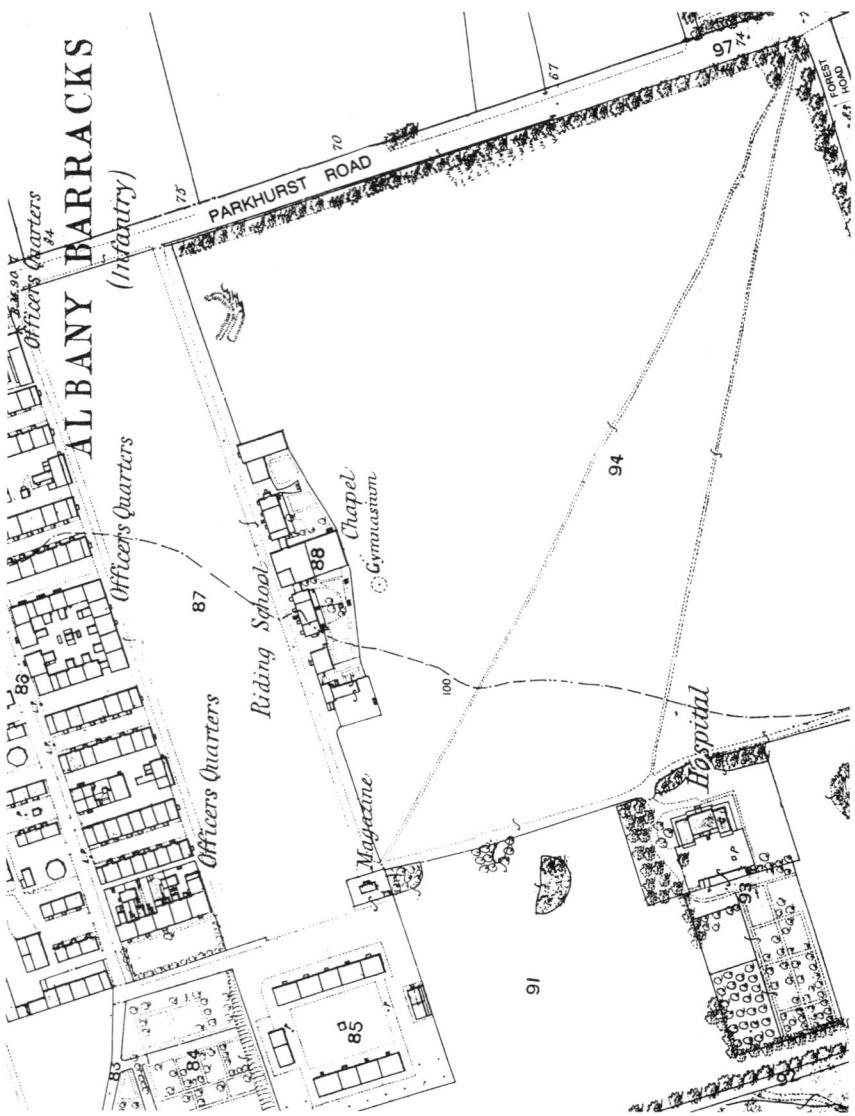

**Figure 11.** Showing the site of the Military Hospital at Albany Barracks. *Courtesy: Ordnance Survey.*

the hospital must have gone with them giving place to the high security prison at Albany.

The hospital at Golden Hill Fort had a shorter life than that at Albany. Details of the building and the history of the fort are given by Cantwell & Sprack in *Solent Papers 2,* from which this brief account is largely taken. The fort was built between 1863 and 1870, as a part of the defences against anticipated hostile attacks from the Continent, - a hexagonal building of two storeys, accommodating 8 officers, 128 other ranks, and with a hospital of 14 beds, on the south aspect of the upper storey, - as is indicated now in explanatory notices for visitors. Cantwell comments that there was a wind pump on the roof above so that the hospital cannot have been a very restful refuge.

Towards the end of the century the fort took on the function of the Western District School of Gunnery; new buildings were put up to the north of the fort and a new hospital was built on the far side of the main road leading from Yarmouth to Colwell and Totland. (See Fig. 12)

In *Shipwrecks of the Wight* J.C. Medland gives an account of the collision on 25th April 1908 in the Solent of the cruiser H.M.S. *Gladiator* and the American Express Mail Liner, *St. Paul*; and mentions that several survivors from the wreck were rescued by soldiers from Fort Victoria and taken to the Golden Hill Fort Hospital and treated there.

In 1912 two of the three blocks comprising the hospital were taken over to be used as quarters and as an officers' mess for the Royal Garrison Artillery. The Army left the Fort and the associated buildings in 1962 and part of the Hospital became a Masonic Lodge.

After the Royal Naval College at Osborne was opened in 1903, two small hospitals were associated with it; both were placed on the opposite, west side of the road from East Cowes to Whippingham; the larger one, termed the Infectious Hospital was made up of four ward blocks plus buildings for administration, admission and discharge (really a gate lodge) and one for disinfection, presumably for clothes and bedding; the other hospital, called the Isolation Hospital was some way off, close to the river and just south of the cemetery and what is now a power station. It was much smaller than the other. The Naval College was closed in 1921; the site of the Upper Hospital and possibly the buildings themselves became for a time the East Cowes Holiday Camp; later it became, and remains, associated with the industrial complex of Saunders Roe and its successors at East Cowes. The buildings which provided the four wards still exist and may be identified on the modern O.S. maps. One supposes that the larger hospital with several wards was available for epidemics

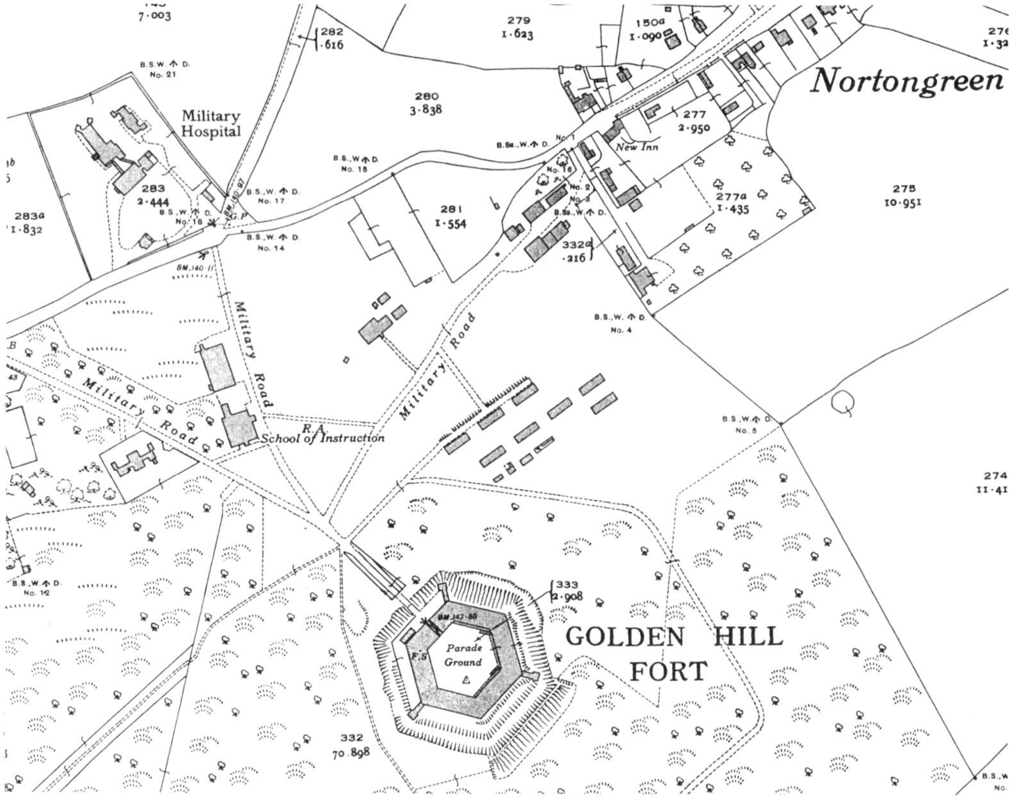

**Figure 12.** The Military Hospital serving Golden Hill Fort. The first hospital was incorporated in the Fort. *Courtesy: Ordnance Survey.*

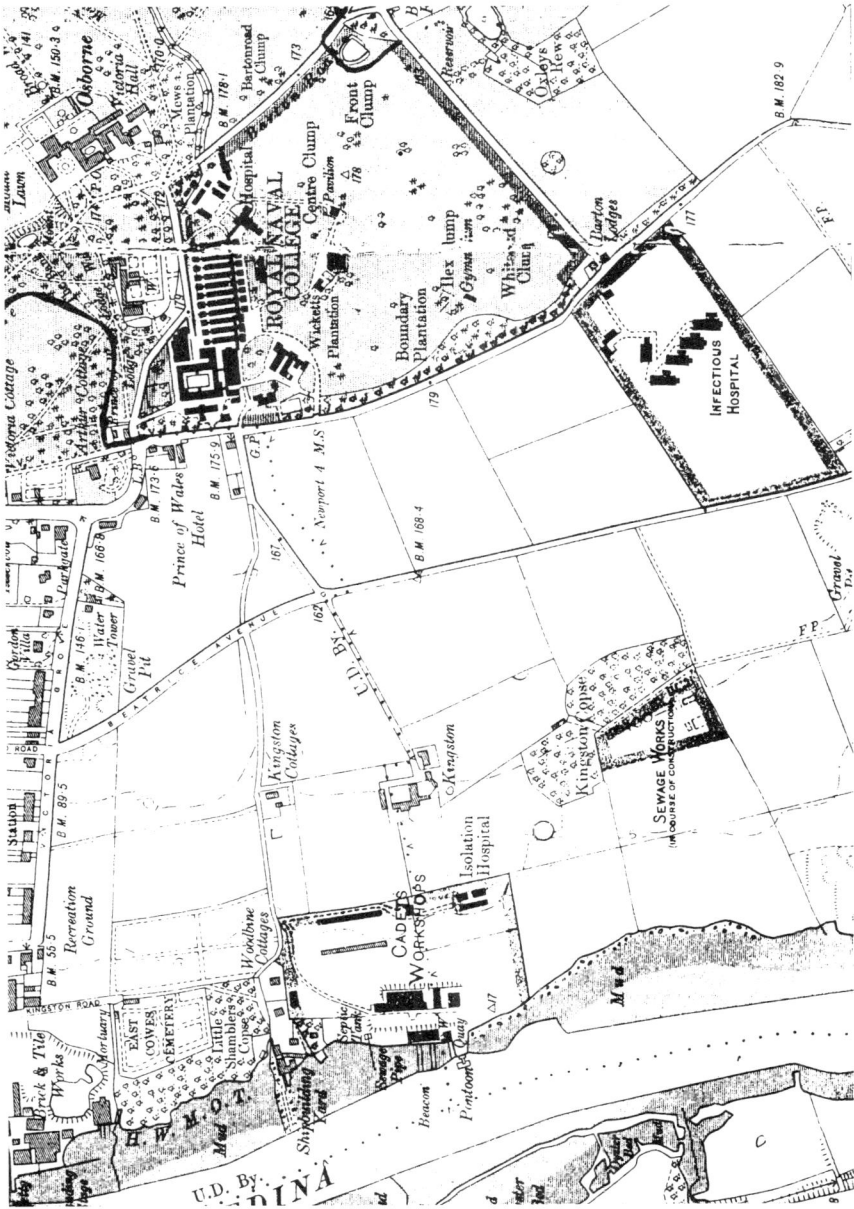

**Figure 13.** Showing the position of the two small hospitals serving the Royal Naval College at Osborne. *Courtesy: Ordnance Survey.*

of infectious diseases which were apparently not uncommon among the Naval cadets who numbered up to 600 at a time; and the smaller one, remote from the college was perhaps intended for Naval personnel possibly returning from stations overseas with communicable diseases.

It was said in the minutes of the Ventnor and Undercliff Hospital about 1925 that the Council was considering purchasing the Osborne Infectious Diseases Hospital; possibly this was the hospital under consideration, - clearly the idea was abandoned.

I am indebted to Mr. A. Freeman of the English Heritage Commission at Osborne for my information about these two small hospitals and for the map. (Fig. 13)

# XI

# PARKHURST PRISON HOSPITAL

The hospitals at Albany Barracks and Parkhurst Prison Hospital, besides their spatial propinquity have it in common that they provided for what may fairly be called a captive clientele exclusively male, and a population officially directed to the Island rather than one born there or coming there from choice.

Parkhurst Prison was initiated about 1840 as a training establishment for boys sentenced to transportation, generally to Australia or New Zealand. About 4,000 boys in all passed through Parkhurst, but after the practice of transportation ceased it became for a time a prison for women; but from 1869 it was exclusively a male prison. The hospital is a separate building within the prison confines; a four storey building with four wards and a number, about 40, of single cells or rooms; it also came to include a radiological department, an operating theatre and a physiotherapy department.

Before the days of the Health Service, the Medical Officers at the prison provided medical care for the prison staff and their families, visiting them at home if needed, and serving in fact as their General Practitioners; and a part of the hospital was set aside for the staff and their families who might need hospital care. In the early days, as mentioned, surgeons came from the adjacent Albany Hospital when needed, to operate upon the inmates of the Prison Hospital; this presumably came to an end when the barracks were closed or empty, and later local consultants were called in as required; Mr. Wilson Harlow during his years at Ryde undertook most of the surgery and was officially appointed as Surgeon to the Hospital, and was followed in this appointment by Mr. Gordon Walker; but other consultants, also visited especially Mr. Philip Grimaldi and Mr. Heckford who did ear, nose and throat work and ophthalmology there. When the other prisons in the neighbourhood, Camphill and Albany came into being, the Parkhurst Hospital served both these as well, so that it dealt with a total population of as many as 2,000; but in addition to its local function it served and continues to serve as a centre within the National Prison Service for psychiatry; prison inmates from all over the country have been brought to Parkhurst for psychiatric treatment and for some time regular sessions for electro-convulsion treatment was held, first at Whitecroft and later within the hospital itself until this form of treatment dropped out of favour. For a short time, about the turn of the century and because of overcrowding in Broadmoor Hospital, while Rampton was being built, a part of Parkhurst Prison was designated as an asylum for the criminally insane; but this was not considered a successful arrangement, in part because of lack of trained staff, and it was soon discontinued.

Another speciality of the Prison Hospital within the Prison Service was the treatment of respiratory disease and especially of Pulmonary Tuberculosis, and considerable numbers of patients from other prisons were moved there for such treatment in the 10 to 15 years after the introduction of the Health Service and before the need for treatment for Tuberculosis became less demanding. During these years a solarium was constructed in order to provide the patients with abundant sunlight and daylight and when the flow of tuberculous patients ceased it was converted into the physiotherapy department.

Five Medical Officers were employed at the hospital, three attached especially to Parkhurst Prison itself and one each for Albany and Camphill, but all co-operating in the work of the hospital; also a number of local General Practitioners used to do some work there on a sessional basis. At all times patients sufficiently seriously ill to require it could be and were moved to hospitals within the region, mostly to the local hospitals on the Island.

All the hospital staff are of course employees of the Home Office as are the rest of the prison staff; the hospital workers are ranked as hospital officers, but a number of them, about one third of the total, having nursing qualifications, and in recent years an increasing number of female trained nurses are working there.

I am grateful to Dr David Cooper who gave me most of the information in this short account of the Prison Hospital.

# PART TWO

*The National Health Service*

# XII

## ADMINISTRATION

On July 5th 1948 the National Health Service (N.H.S.) assumed the management for almost all the hospitals in the country; within their regions hospitals were formed into groups controlled by their Hospital Management Committees (H.M.Cs); on the Island there were two hospital groups - the first comprised all the hospitals save one; the second was the Royal National Hospital which being a specialist hospital and serving mainly patients from the mainland was made a separate group on its own; most of the members of its Management Committee had been on the Board of Management before the appointed day. It remained on its own for a decade and then, with its numbers dwindling and being by then almost entirely for Island patients with only a very few coming from the mainland, it was merged with the other Isle of Wight hospitals. This took place in 1958 at just about the same time as Wessex became a separate region rather than a sub-region of the South-West Metropolitan Region.

The larger group, perhaps rather surprisingly, included so many as 11 hospitals; St. Mary's and Ryde, the general hospitals; the Frank James and Shanklin Cottage Hospitals, and the two other small hospitals in Shanklin, the Arthur Webster Institute and Scio House; Fairlee, the Infectious Diseases Hospital, and the Ventnor and Undercliff Hospital for Infectious Diseases; Longford Sanatorium; the Ashey Smallpox Hospital; and the largest of all, Whitecroft Hospital.

For all these there was now one central management where before there had been about half a dozen more or less independent boards or committees. In this chapter, I endeavour to give an account of this central management and the development of the various aspects of the hospital service, - medicine, surgery, psychiatry, etc., - which necessarily involved all or most of the individual hospitals; and in a subsequent chapter to consider the larger hospitals separately and the way in which they were affected by the evolution of the service.

The H.M.C. managed the hospitals for some 26 years until 1974; the first Chairman was Mr. H.S. Saunders who saw it through the first year and was followed in the chair by Major General Sir H. Roome who carried on for ten years becoming towards the end of that time also Chairman of the R.N.H.

Committee shortly before it merged with the other. Included in the H.M.C. were Dr Wallace, the C.M.O., Dr Dockray, Mr. Leisching, and Mr. O'Donoghue who were all senior consultants on the staff of Ryde or St. Mary's and others who had been on the Management Board of Ryde or of the other hospitals.

The first meeting of the H.M.C. was held before the appointed day (i.e. July 5th 1948) at County Hall; the County Clerk, Mr. Baines, served as Secretary, his offer to do so being gratefully accepted. Later the committee met on one occasion at Frank James Hospital and once at the Ryde Nurses Home, but then settled down to meet at St. Mary's until in 1950 they moved to Clatterford House where offices were available. Several years later a final move took place to what had formerly been the Nurses Home at Whitecroft. Applications had been invited at the start for the posts of Secretary and Finance Officer; there were 206 applications for the former, and 134 for the latter. In October 1948 Mr. J.E. Ray was appointed Secretary and Mr. H. Forshaw Finance Officer. The former left after about a year and Mr. Forshaw for a while seems to have filled both posts. In 1951 Mr. G.F.R. Hardy became Assistant Finance Officer and from the beginning of 1954 he was the Finance Officer and Mr. F.L.W. Eade was Secretary. These two remained in their posts, in effect the professional heads of the administration, up to the close of this phase of the N.H.S. in 1974. Major General M. Hext took over from Sir. H. Roome in 1959 and like him served for about a decade, and then Mrs. T. Margham became Chairman of the H.M.C. for its remaining years. The Chairmen were in all cases also members of the Regional Board.

There were of course a number of sub-committees including medical and nursing sub-committees. These were advisory and not executive; the Medical Committee met monthly and included all consultants. In those early years consultants did not expect to have their work interrupted by committee meetings and at first the Medical Committee met at 8.30 in the evening once a month; there was at least one occasion on which the meeting continued until 11 p.m.

There were in 1948 two farms, - at St. Mary's and Whitecroft - and the Central Farm Committee, a sub-committee of the H.M.C. dealt with these, and they were evidently looked upon quite seriously. Early in 1949 the H.M.C. agreed to spend £1,000 on a dairy herd to provide milk for St. Mary's, and Dolly, BlueBird, Maisie, Jonah (!), Sally, Daisy and Susanne took up residence at St. Mary's and their yield of milk was duly reported each quarter to the H.M.C., as was that of the Whitecroft herd; pigs and poultry were kept at both hospitals (poultry also at Longford) and swill was collected from the kitchens; at Ryde swill had hitherto been sold locally and had brought the hospital £60 a year, but now was passed onto the piggeries at St. Mary's. Vegetables were grown at both hospitals, also at Fairlee and Longford. The staff for these activities included farm bailiffs at St. Mary's and Whitecroft; half a dozen garden and farm labourers at Whitecroft; a gardener, three labourers and a dairy maid at St. Mary's, and ten gardeners in all at the other hospitals.

At Ventnor in the other group, pigs, poultry and often geese were kept and there were large gardens which supplied much of the hospital's vegetables, apples and soft fruit; there was a farm bailiff and head gardener and a number of other gardeners.

In 1953 however the Ministry decided that hospitals were not to continue farming or market gardening (garden and farm products supplied to the hospital's kitchens were always debited at the market rates to catering accounts) and farms were abandoned and the stock sold off; a head gardener remained on the staff at Whitecroft and St. Mary's; in each of which there were fairly extensive grounds; and several other gardeners were retained full-time or part-time at other hospitals.

It is convenient at this point to mention also the maintenance staff which for the whole group included two engineers in charge; a foreman/carpenter, and five carpenters; four brick layers and four brick layers' labourers; three electricians; one painter; four plumbers and fitters; and two and a half labourers.


The accommodation for infectious diseases was an early concern of the H.M.C.; the hospital at Ventnor (the Undercliff Isolation Hospital - not of course the R.N.H.) had been under-used for many years and Fairlee Hospital - the only one now used for infectious diseases on the Island, - was also usually lightly occupied, as is inevitable in a hospital which deals with sporadic epidemics. Dr Wallace was asked to report on the situation and to consider the possibility of using the Ventnor Hospital alone for the whole Island and converting Fairlee Hospital to some other use. He reported that additional building would be needed at Ventnor and that given that it would be possible to use it as the only Island isolation hospital, but it was out of the way and barely suitable in other ways and he did not think it would be a wise measure; this opinion was not disputed and that was the end of the Ventnor and Undercliff Hospital as such.

After the Poliomyelitis epidemic of 1950 there was rather little demand, (which is not to say there was none at all) for beds for treating infectious diseases in isolation. It was not long before, on the recommendation of the Medical Advisory Committee, half of the beds at Fairlee were taken over for the 'chronic sick'.

Hospitals and beds for the treatment of Tuberculosis, especially respiratory Tuberculosis, were in demand in the early years of the service and the hospitals and sanatoria were full and had waiting lists for admission; the rapid changes in this situation during the first decade of the N.H.S. was due, as already indicated, to the advent of effective drug treatment; it was only by chance that this coincided with the development of the N.H.S.. Longford Hospital as previously described was used for the Island patients and from 1948 Dr Easton was its Chest Physician and Superintendent at the sanatorium; the Catherine Bowen Home built in the grounds of Longford was available for children, but after the war it was in poor repair and was considered inadequate and in 1952, after it had been done up, it was used to provide beds for adults, and the few children who needed hospital treatment went to the White House Hospital at Milford. Before long with the use of effective drugs the problem of beds for Tuberculosis (on the Island anyhow) disappeared; and in 1955 Longford Hospital ceased to be a sanatorium; Dr Easton moved to an appointment in Scotland; and mentally handicapped women and girls were moved from St. Mary's to Longford, leaving more and better accommodation for the men; Longford Hospital was thereafter managed in conjunction with Whitecroft and the consultants there were in charge of the patients.

The senior medical staff were at the time of the take-over few in number compared with modern times. There were three Consultant Surgeons, and one Orthopaedic Surgeon who was graded at first as a Senior Hospital Medical Officer, - becoming a Consultant later; he had at the start the support of a Senior Orthopaedic Consultant, Mr. Ellis who took the place of Mr. Langston and who visited Ryde Hospital at first fortnightly and later at longer intervals; and later again the Consultant in post, Mr. E. Smythe had the help of a senior assistant.

The three surgeons were Mr. Leisching who before 1948 had concerned himself especially with Orthopaedic surgery, and had organised a mobile physiotherapy unit: Mr. F. Wilson Harlow, author of a textbook on *Surgery For Nurses,* well known and widely used for a time: and Mr. Gaynor who like his colleagues worked at both general hospitals but also had a particular association with Shanklin Cottage Hospital; he died in the early years of the N.H.S. and his place was taken by Mr. V. Gordon Walker.

Dr V. Clark and Dr Phoebe Harvey were the consultant anaesthetists and several G.P.s provided additional sessions, in particular Dr Bruce, Dr John Mackett, and Dr Hooker.

There were two physicians who shared the work at Ryde and St. Mary's; the need for an additional physician was soon recognised, but it was not until 1950 that Dr J.C. Harland was appointed. Arriving on the Island, he was almost immediately summoned to the Obstetric Ward at St. Mary's, being the only consultant available on the Island at that time to assist in a difficult delivery - the Consultant Obstetrician being temporarily at sea (literally); a somewhat unexpected and possibly embarrassing baptism; but with the help and support of the ward sister, a highly experienced midwife, a happy outcome was achieved. Dr Harland like the other physicians worked at both hospitals but tended to do more at St. Mary's and there also for some years he had charge of a large number of chronic sick patients in the Lower Hospital. Dr Dockray and Dr Firman-Edwards also worked at both hospitals; it has been said that they were reluctant to work at what had been the Infirmary, but I think this is quite untrue and unfair; both practised in Ryde and had worked at the hospital there for many years and for that and other reasons they tended to continue working more there than at Newport, but certainly both of them had patients at Newport and were perfectly ready to do their share of work there.

At Ventnor, Dr Miller besides being Superintendent was Consultant Chest Physician for the Island; he had access, if needed, to a couple of beds in St. Mary's, and he supervised the work at Longford visiting there weekly so long as it remained a Tuberculosis sanatorium. He had one senior assistant and two resident juniors, - another was added when more surgery was tackled.

At Whitecroft Dr Gordon Brown had a Deputy Superintendent, Dr Wood who had been there from about 1932, and one junior. Dr Davies-Jones who was the retired Superintendent for a time did a few out-patient sessions chiefly with children. Dr Gordon Brown was the Consultant Psychiatrist for the Island as had been his predecessors.

Mr. O'Donoghue was the Obstetrician and Gynaecologist, working at St. Mary's. Dr Barker had been Radiologist for several years before the N.H.S. and was now appointed the full-time Consultant Radiologist for the Island. Mr. Heckford also had been on the Island a long time, being Consultant Ophthalmic Surgeon since 1931, but the Island had not until now had a resident Consultant E.N.T. Surgeon and Mr. Philip Grimaldi was appointed to that post. Dr Thornton and Dr Darmady had been Visiting Consultant Pathologists since before the war, Dr Thornton retired soon after the war and Dr Darmady became Director of Pathology at Portsmouth, the service there incorporating the

Pathology services for the Island where Dr Dobson was appointed a Consultant Pathologist; he covered the work at Ventnor also, visiting there once a week, and a technician was appointed at Ventnor; there were of course a number of technicians at Ryde laboratory and a small laboratory was opened at St. Mary's.

Resident staff were also few compared with later years. At Ryde there were at first two residents, H.S. and H.P., who had between them to cover the Casualty department and each other's time off duty. Before long a second H.S. was added for the duties in the Orthopaedic Wards and Casualty Department. At Newport similarly a House Surgeon and a House Physician were later supplemented by an Obstetric House Surgeon and a casualty House Surgeon. In 1951 the H.M.C. decreed that an H.P. or H.S. should have one half day a week off duty and one weekend in three off from 4 p.m. on Friday to Sunday (presumably in practice Monday morning). One must suppose that at that time there was no national or regional standard; no doubt other hospital groups also regarded this as an adequate arrangement and it is only fair to acknowledge that demands were very much less heavy in those days.

In the cottage hospitals General Practitioners in the locality provided a service and worked a duty rota so that one was always available if needed; some casualties were treated at the Frank James Hospital. In return for their services G.P.s had the right to admit patients to the beds in his hospital; later each of them was used to supplement, especially, the surgical services of the general hospitals.

At Frank James Hospital G.P.s and Consultants did regular operating sessions and later for a time there was a session in Orthopaedic surgery and in Gynaecology; and at Shanklin, the E.N.T. Consultant did a regular list of tonsillectomies and one of the practitioners functioning first as a Clinical Assistant and later as a Medical Assistant did a list of general surgery.

The Obstetric service was developed at St. Mary's; here the move of the chronic sick patients from the Infirmary to the Lower Hospital liberated some space for other things and Gynaecological and Obstetric wards were quickly set up in block A; in the course of time the upper floor came to be purely for Gynaecology and the lower floor for Midwifery. The small ward - Carisbrooke Ward - which had been previously the Obstetric Ward was after this used for various purposes. The Obstetric accommodation was increased to 35 which permitted the establishment of a school for midwifery. So early as 1949 there was a call for an Obstetric Flying Squad, but this was never established. In 1952 the Consultant Obstetrician, Mr. O'Donoghue, and the local Medical Committee agreed in principle that a General Practitioner wing at St. Mary's, independent of the Midwifery Training School, but under the general supervision of the consultant, should be set up; but this did not get further at the time and several years later in 1959 it was again recommended, but without any immediate action. The accommodation for midwifery was always regarded as somewhat unsatisfactory; among other difficulties all the traffic from the surgical wards to the theatre and back had to pass through this department. In 1964 Mr. O'Donoghue retired and later Mr. W. Edwards was appointed Obstetrician and Gynaecologist, but it was still a decade before the large new Obstetric Department was opened at St. Mary's.

The Orthopaedic surgery services were from the start naturally associated with the Casualty Department, and this had initially, both at Ryde and at Newport, to share common accommodation with the Out-patient Department. By 1954 there was a full-time consultant in Orthopaedic Surgery and the department then and ever since has maintained an association with the Lord Mayor Treloar Hospital at Alton. In 1954 a Casualty House Surgeon was appointed at Ryde who would also serve in the Orthopaedic Ward. Later, a second Assistant Casualty Officer was appointed to the staff. The Orthopaedic beds were on the upper floors at Ryde, and later wholly in Beatrice Ward which was in two parts, one for men and one for ladies and was conveniently close to the theatre; but in the second half of the 1950s especially there was repeated call for more Orthopaedic accommodation, and along with this for more physiotherapy and more sessions by the Physical Medicine Consultant, Dr Saville, who came over from Portsmouth; and also for a Rehabilitation Unit and a Department of Daily Living. The shortage of beds was eased for a time by the transfer of a number of convalescent orthopaedic patients to the R.N.H. at Ventnor where, surgical sessions being ended by the close of 1958, there were now beds readily available. Another arrangement was to borrow a few beds in the Military Hospital at Albany Barracks close to St. Mary's Hospital and this was organised by the Regional Board. Despite these measures at the end of 1961 most orthopaedic patients waited more than a year for their planned operation and many more than two years; it was arranged that extra operating sessions each week should be worked at the Frank James Hospital and also Shanklin Cottage Hospital; more beds were made available at each of these hospitals; and after six months a considerable improvement had been achieved and 24 extra operating sessions had been carried out at the Frank James Hospital; the waiting list was reduced from 189 to 109.

During most of this phase of the N.H.S., Casualty Departments functioned both at Ryde and at St. Mary's; at Ryde a new Out-patient Department was built very early on in the Health Service and improvements were made in the layout of the Casualty Department. In St. Mary's the two departments continued to have a common entrance, but in the 1960s additional building provided a new Out-patient waiting hall and three new sets of consulting rooms. Apart from considerations of space, shortage of staff made the casualty service difficult to maintain and in 1970 at St. Mary's it had for some time to be closed at the weekends and at night, and operate only in 'office hours', that is from 8 a.m. to 6 p.m. on five days a week.

It was in association with the Orthopaedic and Physical Medicine Departments that a school for spastic and other disabled children was started and was housed in the building immediately opposite the Forest Road which had formerly been first a porter's lodge and reception wards and later provided accommodation for a bailiff and others; it now became known as Forest Side School and flourished for several years; the construction of the relief road at the approach from Cowes to Newport involved the loss of land at the south-west corner of the hospital estate, a good part of which had been known as the cricket ground, and also the demolition of this building and the cultivated land immediately around it. The school moved, after consideration, to Watergate, and to the disappointment of the hospital service lost its connection with St. Mary's. The H.M.C. was moved to express its regret that at the opening of the new school at Watergate no representative of the Health Service was invited. About the same time a hostel for handicapped children, Castle View, was opened close to Polars Blind Home on Staplers.

In 1973 a second Consultant in Orthopaedic Surgery, Mr. de Belder was appointed.


Victoria Ward at Ryde was to remain for the whole of the 26 years of the H.M.C.'s existence the principal, - and indeed almost the only ward available for children; at the beginning of this time, i.e. the start of the Health Service, Paediatrics was becoming a speciality, although it was a decade before any specialist Paediatrician was to be resident on the Island. In 1951 it was agreed that children admitted to Ryde would be under the care of Dr E. Firman-Edwards, and that Dr Moseley, Paediatrician at Portsmouth, would visit regularly to give advice or to take over a patient when necessary. Visiting was to be allowed every evening for child patients - at first as a trial for six months. In 1958 Victoria Ward had to be closed for alterations; children with acute illnesses were then to be admitted when necessary to the medical wards at Ryde or Newport. Later in that year Dr Firman-Edwards retired, and Dr Miller became the first children's specialist to reside on the Island; he shared the duties with Dr Moseley and he also stood in for him at Portsmouth and did a session there; this was in addition to his work as a General Physician. The separation of the Children's Ward from the Obstetric Department was repeatedly deplored through these years, but it remained so until a later phase in the hospital's life. This was one aspect of the disadvantages of two general hospitals on the Island where there was really only scope for one. The two Consultant Physicians on the Island were heard to say that the only time they met each other was on Wootton Bridge when one was travelling from Ryde to Newport and the other from Newport to Ryde.

The Act of 1948 had imposed upon county councils the obligation to provide residential accommodation for old people in need of care, but not in need of hospital nursing; this provision was specified in Part Three of the Act and hence the homes came to be known, - and are often still known - as Part Three Homes. Several such homes were set up on the Island over the years, the first one being St. Lawrence Dene and Underwath; others followed - Inver House in Bembridge, Elmdon in Shanklin, Osborne Cottage in East Cowes, possibly the only Part Three Home in the country established in what had formerly been the regular residence of members of the Royal Family, Polars in Newport where a home for the blind was also provided; and later Steephill House in St. Lawrence formerly the nurses home of the R.N.H., and the Gouldings in Freshwater. Patients suitable for such homes were gradually moved from St. Mary's and from Whitecroft to the homes which of course took residents from the general population also. When this was done there was still a large group of old people left in St. Mary's, and in Whitecroft, who were not ill in any way that, in the state of medicine at that time, was thought likely to benefit from the services of a Consultant Surgeon or Physician, but who did need nursing care; that is, more care than could be expected at a residential home.

Such patients, recruited from the general population on the recommendation of their General Practitioners, or from the medical and surgical wards of the general hospitals, having been admitted to these general wards and thereafter failing to recover sufficiently to be discharged, made up here as elsewhere a large proportion of the whole hospital population. They came to occupy what was remembered by the Island population as the Workhouse, now known as the Lower Hospital, where there were four large wards for them; to these, later, was added one ward at Fairlee no longer needed for infectious diseases. Among these patients ladies always outnumbered men by more than two to one; they were under the supervision of a Consultant Physician and in general it was not expected that they would be discharged, - although a few made sufficient progress to be transferred to their homes. These wards also included a number of younger patients, more or less severely disabled with incurable illnesses such as Multiple Sclerosis, severe Rheumatoid Arthritis and other long lasting illnesses. For these unfortunate patients who needed comprehensive nursing, there was for many years no better provision. When the writer took over the Geriatric service in 1963 there were still about 10% of 160 beds occupied by such young patients all under 60, and some of them still in their 30s.

In 1951 the Medical Advisory Committee urged that Physiotherapy and Almoning services for these chronic sick should be improved; and that the use of the garrets (i.e. the top floor) for patients should cease and that better arrangements for admission and discharge to Part Three Homes should be made. By 1952 still 18 patients considered suitable for Part Three Homes remained in St. Mary's where the wards remained full.

A large proportion of the whole number of these people suffered from what is now called, - or sometimes miscalled, - Alzheimer's Disease. The same was true of many of the older patients in Whitecroft Hospital. Such patients all over the country had tended to accumulate in hospitals or infirmaries and mental hospitals run by the county councils and were the cause of the indifferent reputation which these hospitals tended to have, always the poor relations of the voluntary hospitals; and that was because they had, without choice, to accept such patients. The Geriatric service, - inchoate at the time of origin of the N.H.S. - was gradually accepted by the administration of the N.H.S. and slowly brought about some improvement, so that in later years to an increasing extent it would be recognised that a proportion at least of the aged could be treated successfully and discharged and that measures to prevent premature invalidity were possible and worthwhile.

Here the Geriatric service began in 1961, when Dr Penman was appointed after the death of Dr Dockray; he was directed to initiate a service, having at the same time a share of the general medical work and doing his stint of dealing with medical emergencies; there was at that time still only one H.P. at St. Mary's to deal with all the medical cases and all patients in the Lower Hospital; moreover Physiotherapy and Occupational Therapy services in the Lower Hospital were extremely slender for many years to come. Dr Penman soon produced a report upon the wards and staff showing how much more could be used; but it was not until he had moved on, that a second House Physician was appointed and several years later the House Physician's job in the Geriatric Department became the first component of a two year appointment, which also included work in the Paediatric, Obstetric and Psychiatric divisions. The Geriatric wards were 'upgraded' and improved and a new reception ward was built (see below) and in time further additions of staff came about.

The Ophthalmic Department and the E.N.T. Department remained at the County Hospital although clinics were held at Newport; and Mr. Philip Grimaldi operated regularly at Shanklin Cottage Hospital and Dr Crosskey for a time did a regular session of Tonsillectomies at the Frank James Hospital. Dental surgery had been available at both hospitals before the N.H.S. and it continued to be so, though reading through the minutes one cannot but feel that the Department of Dentistry was rather pushed around with many changes of location.

Nursing staff at Ryde did not have to undergo any major re-arrangement after the start of the Health Service; the King George VI Nurses Home had been opened just before the war and a Nurse Training School had been initiated also before the war. There were problems about accommodation for student nurses. Two houses were involved, - the Towers in Partlands Avenue which was leased and was in use in July 1948 and which, at that time and for a while afterwards, the H.M.C. sought to purchase; agreement with the proprietors could not be reached and there was talk of compulsory purchase; however in 1950 it was decided to give up the Towers and a lease was obtained of St. Wilfred's, a house somewhat further away from the hospital, though not very far, which was to be used as a residence. Victor House in Partlands Avenue had been purchased before 1948 by the hospital and £5,000 of the total sum of £15,000 had been paid and this served as the actual training school.

St. Mary's Hospital was now to develop into a general hospital. In 1948 there had been 17 nurses there plus a number of nursing orderlies; by April 1952 there were 82 nurses, although 10 fewer nursing orderlies. Miss Roker was the first Matron, in office on the appointed day; she was succeeded by Miss Cooper, and in 1952 by Miss Sylvia White who continued until 1969, the last Matron of St. Mary's. In 1949 a training school for State Enrolled Nurses was opened and in 1950 in a report the King Edward Fund commented that St. Mary's gave exceptionally good opportunities for the training of assistant nurses.

Shortage of nurses was a problem from time to time in every hospital. In

1952 the appointment of non-resident nurses was encouraged, since there was a lack of residential accommodation, but student nurses were required to remain resident. Before the Health Service ward orderlies had been appointed when nurses were not available; again in 1963 nursing auxiliaries filled the gap and made up 25% of nursing staff in the region; a plan for their duties and instruction was issued; introductory talks included those on courtesy, taking messages, and relationship with trained nurses and others, - an echo perhaps of 1849. In 1955 the G.N.C. had approved of the association of the R.N.H. and Ryde for nurse training; one year was to be spent at the R.N.H. and two at Ryde. Numbers both of patients and nurses at the R.N.H. were dwindling soon after this and the number of nurses involved in this training was small; nevertheless some of them achieved an excellent record and high positions in the nursing world. In 1961 a further report from the G.N.C. confirmed the continuation of nursing schools at Ryde, St. Mary's and Whitecroft with various recommendations. Fairlee Hospital was to participate in the training, but not the Cottage Hospitals or Longford. The appointment of 10 additional nurses in 1953 within the group was approved, but their salaries had to come from the existing allotment! And in 1960 the H.M.C. again sought a substantial increase in the senior nursing staff in the group by 9 sisters and 7 staff nurses.

In 1965 the appointment of a Group Tutor was recommended and the training of nurses was to be carried on at St. Mary's, Ryde and in the acute wards at Whitecroft.

Another nurses' home was built about 1966 and in 1969 a new Nurse Training School built at St. Mary's was opened by the Governor of the Island, Lord Louis Mountbatten. The year before this the Isle of Wight Society of Nurses had been founded. Meanwhile, the whole system of nursing administration in the Health Service had been altered by the introduction of the 'Salmon Scheme'. In 1967 the H.M.C. agreed that the Island should be chosen as a group for a trial of this scheme. However, by the time the trial got under way, it was already quite apparent to the medical and nursing professions that the scheme was to be implemented nationally, and the outcome of the trial was a foregone conclusion. When the necessary changes in the nursing administration locally were expounded to the Medical Advisory Committee by the Group Secretary it is fair to comment that, when the question was put 'Is the success of this trial already established in the minds of those who are judging it?', the diplomatic answer was 'Naturally we should not embark upon a trial of this nature if we did not expect it to succeed'.

It is perhaps of some interest to give figures of the cost of the hospital service at the beginning and the end of this phase, a period of about 25 years.

I give here a brief summary of the figures for the first full year 1949-50 and the last 1973-74. These were the estimates agreed upon and submitted by the treasurer to the H.M.C. We have to remember that the value of money changed considerably during this period; according to Whitaker's Almanac the purchasing power of the pound in your pocket declined by about two thirds between 1949 and 1974 and it has declined about a further five fold since then so that a pound in 1949 would have bought approximately what £15 buys now or what £3 bought in 1973.

## Table 2 . Annual Expenditure

| Item | 1949-1950 | 1973-74 |
|---|---|---|
| Medical Salaries | 4,031 * | 58,200 * |
| Nursing Salaries | 74,107 | 960,400 |
| All other Salaries | 82,004 | 702,040 |
| Central Administration | 13,425 | 71,300 |
| Drugs, Dressing & Appliances | 16,814 | 157,750 |
| Provisions | 42,207 | 122,000 |
| Fuel, Light, Power & Water | 22,368 | 94,600 |
| Rates & Rent | 29,700 | 45,200 |
| Uniforms & Clothing | 4,928 | 16,100 |
| Laundry & Cleaning | 2,116 | 16,750 |
| Total (including items not tabulated above) | 308,419 | 2,471,400 |

*The salaries of doctors above the rank of House-man and SHO were paid by the Regional Board, not the H.M.C.

# XIII

# THE HOSPITALS

## ——————— *The Royal Isle of Wight County Hospital* ———————

Ryde Hospital was always handicapped in its development by lack of space into which it could expand. It was, and is, bounded on three sides by roads, any space on the fourth, south side, being limited to a narrowing wedge as two roads, Swanmore Road and West Street converge. The nurses home built in a very pleasant garden had good space around it, but was too far away to serve for any extension of the main hospital, although near enough to be convenient as a nurses' home.

A house in Swanmore Road, adjacent to the hospital, was bought by the H.M.C. and served for an extension of the X-ray Department, with a flat upstairs for a resident doctor; and later a second adjacent house allowed further extension; but to get more space, accommodation had to be found in nearby Partlands Avenue. Ultimately, three houses in line were required; these three were joined by covered corridors and served as a physiotherapy centre for Ryde. When a new Nurse Training School came into operation at St. Mary's the training school at Ryde closed, but that house was added to the ancillary departments of the hospital. The upstairs of these houses provided a flat for the resident medical staff, a nurse's flat and accommodation for ambulance staff; all these, like the physiotherapy centre itself, were connected to the hospital switchboard.

Ryde Hospital continued throughout this phase and indeed until 1990 to provide the main Accident and Emergency Department; the problem for the administration was to make this separate from the Out-patient Department, - which in the first place had shared accommodation with it; the Out-patient entrance at that time had been in Milligan Street and in the masonry above the closed door, one can still make out the words 'Out-patient Entrance'. Plans for a new Out-patient Department and for improvement of the Casualty Department were produced in 1950. Before that, hutted accommodation for out-patients had been considered. Now, however, some rooms occupied hitherto by nursing staff on the north side of the ground floor were converted into an Out-patient Department and about the same time rooms in the front of the hospital, which had been part of the resident staff quarters, were re-arranged, giving an entrance hall and a sitting-dining room for consultants on the south side of the main entrance. On the north side was the telephone switchboard and beyond that the dispensary, later called the pharmacy.

About this time the hospital was invited and agreed to take over the work of the old Ryde dispensary, which for several years now had been situated close to the hospital in the angle between Swanmore Road and West Street, now the Ryde headquarters of the Red Cross.

Work on the new Out-patient Department and the construction of an entrance to it from West Street and also the upgrading of the Casualty Department continued until 1957; during this time also, the hot water system for the hospital was renovated and cubiculising (or later cubicularisation!) of the wards was begun. Meanwhile the ground floor of the Milligan Convalescent Home was taken over as the headquarters of the Records Department and as a Secretary's office; and on the first floor there was a dining-room for the nursing staff, also used for some other purposes, including for a time, meetings of the Medical Advisory Committee. Further improvements in the Out-patient Department were to come in 1960.

From time to time, the minutes of the Hospital Management Committee and the County Hospital House Committee mention a roof garden at Ryde, proposed and possibly planned; I have been unable to find anyone who recalls the real thing and I do not think it can ever have come into being. In 1972-73 the X-ray Department was further enlarged and the Casualty Department, now to be known as the Accident and Emergency Department, was also re-designed and improved. In-filling of the available space around the Out-patient Department provided more consulting rooms and offices for medical secretaries and others and a way was made through from the Out-patient Department to the Records Office and the rest of the old Milligan Block. The old lift, built about the beginning of the First World War, needed replacement and a new one was built, the old shaft providing space for new storage cupboards.

Private work had always been carried out at the County Hospital to a modest extent and at the start of the N.H.S. two categories of private wards were generally allowed to be used in hospitals; single wards, and amenity beds which would be small wards with two or three patients only. At Ryde there were eight and later nine single wards in the building named in memory of a former Treasurer and Chairman, Aubrey Wickham; these were on the first floor at the north end of the hospital, more or less over the Casualty Department and where formerly had been the wards for infectious diseases. They were available for private patients, but it was always agreed that in case of necessity, for whatever precise reason, a single room might be taken for other patients, and this was occasionally put into practice; for example, when boys had to be admitted from the Borstal Institute; this principle prevailed both before and after the National Health Service. It may be mentioned here that small numbers of private beds were also available in Shanklin Cottage Hospital and at the Frank James Hospital. There were never any at St. Mary's despite repeated requests that there should be a few, especially in the Obstetric Department.

## St. Mary's Hospital

At the start of the N.H.S. there was still a Lay Superintendent or Master, Mr. Bennett, at St. Mary's who had authority over and responsibility for the non-medical and non-nursing components of the hospital as well as Forest House; his assistant, Mr. Hunt remained for a time after he retired, and became the assistant to Mr. J. Keech who was appointed Hospital Secretary to St. Mary's in 1950. From the start, and indeed for several years before 1948 it had been recognised that St. Mary's would have to be the site of the principal general hospital on the Island. This was propounded by the C.M.O., Dr Fairley in 1944 and was reiterated from time to time. The idea was of course challenged by the medical staff at Ryde, but I think that after 1948 there was never any serious doubt in anyone's mind about it. However, several years later when it came to actual planning of the new district hospital the consultants collectively proposed that the Whitecroft site should be preferred for development and they pressed the point with some enthusiasm; their opinion, however, was unsupported by the H.M.C. or the Regional Board and was quickly rejected by the Ministry.

It may be of interest here to recall a much earlier suggestion of an alternative site for the development of the Island's hospitals. In 1928, when Ryde Hospital committee was looking for more room, Sir Guise Morris suggested that Ryde Hospital should be abandoned, and a new hopsital set up on the Westwood Estate, on the North side of Lushington Hill. This suggestion was immediately rejected, but it is diverting to speculate for a moment on the idea: the estate, which then may have reached east-west roughly from top to bottom of Lushington Hill and north-south from Lushington Hill to Brock's Copse Lane: would have been large enough for the whole hospital complex: it was central - near both Ryde, Newport and East Cowes and not that far from Cowes; and it was close to the ferries at East Cowes and Fishbourne. It might have made a quite considerable difference to the whole evolution of the Island.

In the early days of the N.H.S. the wards at St. Mary's were given names of different villages or districts on the Island, and Womens' Institutes in these localities undertook to adopt the wards and to take a special interest in them. There were two exceptions to these names. The first, Rookwood Ward was 'adopted' by the prison staff at Parkhurst. The name 'Rookwood' was an authorised euphemism for Parkhurst Prison, rather in the same way that 'Forest House' was adopted as an alternative name to the Workhouse; it meant that letters could be written or reference made to residence without using the term Parkhurst Prison; this was how Rookwood Ward acquired its name, which remains. The second case later in the hospital's history was Hassall Ward named after the founder of the Royal National Hospital at Ventnor, this ward to some extent taking the place of the R.N.H. after it was closed.

Before it could function as an adequate general hospital, many additions and alterations were needed, and all were aware of this: requests, demands and plans were made by the Regional Board, the Hospital Management Committee and the Medical Advisory Committee from 1949 onwards; but money for building was always limited and until much later and in a different phase of the hospital's life, it was more or less accepted that additions had to be provided piecemeal; and the pressure of needs together with limitation of the funds led, from time to time, to curious plans which happily were abandoned before they were seriously worked out; - such was the Regional Board's plan in 1968 to have all general medicine and surgery at St. Mary's and to use Ryde for Ophthalmology, E.N.T. surgery, and Geriatrics.

When the district hospital was eventually planned, on paper, the Regional Board suggested that the Lower or South Hospital should be demolished, the geriatric patients accommodated there being moved to the North Hospital! The first date given for the completion of the new hospital was 1971!

The first new building at St. Mary's was the one-storey Out-patient department and X-ray room north of the porter's lodge; these were available in 1950 and were soon extended to include rooms for a chest clinic; over the years there were many additions to this building, partly in the form of Portakabins and partly by rather more permanent buildings.

The amount of work required in the chest clinic declined gradually and its rooms were used at times for physiotherapy, for dentistry and for radiotherapy. The records department obtained a more permanent and enlarged foothold there in the 1970s and the X-ray department was considerably enlarged. An earlier improvement had been the building of a new waiting hall for out-patients separating them from casualties, together with three further sets of consulting rooms which gave accommodation for the increasing number of clinics held there.

The hospital pharmacy, or dispensary as it was at first called, was at the start housed in a hut attached to the Upper Hospital; during 1952 the need for enlargement was obvious and a 'prefab' building was put up on the north side of the drive opposite St. Catherine's Ward and served right up to the opening of the new St. Mary's. An extension of this building provided three flats for resident doctors and another flat above the old lodge was similarly used for a time; throughout the years of the H.M.C. this porter's lodge housed the switchboard; the rooms extending eastward from the lodge, originally intended for the reception of patients being admitted to the H of I, were used as offices for the hospital secretary, his assistant and his clerk and the Social Services and for a time the Lady Almoner attached to the hospital.

The increase in nursing staff of course led to a need for more residential accommodation; at the start nurses had resident quarters in the middle block of the Upper Hospital on its upper floors; the southern wing provided a flat, at first for the matron, later for the assistant matron, and some offices; the north wing which lay over the nurses' dining room and the kitchens for the Upper Hospital provided quarters for sisters and nurses. In the Lower Hospital (or H of I) rooms were provided over the boardroom and the east end of the main building was now used as a nurse training school. In 1952 a new nurses' home was built, a long one-storey building looking south-east, to the east of the Upper Hospital, providing rooms for about twenty nurses. This building of course is still in use, though not for nurses.

Later the nurse training school was established at St. Mary's, - a new building below this nurses' home with lecture rooms, library, laboratory, etc., and this was opened by Lord Louis Mountbatten, in 1969 - who gave it the name of the 'Royal Isle of Wight School of Nursing'; also a further nurses' home was built below the training school, as mentioned above.

In the early years of the H.M.C. all the wards at St. Mary's were heated, and hot water supplied, from individual coke ovens and boilers for each ward. The boiler house lying to the east of the Lower Hospital near the gate in from Dodnor Lane supplied heating for the main Lower Hospital buildings and steam for the laundry and the kitchen there.

The existing boiler had been installed about 1920 and Bill Shepard has given an entertaining account and picture of how it was hauled up from the quay to the hospital. Now over about two decades the heating system was brought up to date. Two new oil-fired boilers semi-automatically controlled were installed in place of the old one and the heating and steam extended to the whole of the Upper Hospital as well as to the outlying parts of the Lower Hospital, the Out-patient department, etc.

Much had to be done for the Upper Hospital especially for those wards which had regularly to accept emergency admissions, and for the theatre, the layout and ancillary rooms for which had to be extended and modernised. In 1959 there was still no lift for the upper wards, which housed all the medical patients; all patients unable to walk upstairs had to be carried up. During 1960 a major scheme of upgrading was undertaken for the medical and surgical wards, familiarly known as Upper B and Lower B; a lift was provided in the centre block of the hospital and the whole of the four wards were to some degree modernised and their toilet facilities improved. This work lasted over some months and during that time the medical wards were moved down to one of the separate blocks on the west side of the Lower Hospital which had been vacated when the mentally handicapped women and girls moved from St. Mary's to Longford. These were old fashioned buildings, one ward occupying two floors with about 30 beds. Each floor was divided into a number of rooms, there was no lift, all patients and meals had to be carried upstairs; there was one bathroom on the ground floor; to provide an adequate medical service over a period of several months on such a ward must have been extremely difficult.

Once this work was completed, the medical and surgical wards were far better able to deal with the emergency and planned admissions which were required; about this time too a medical registrar was appointed for the first time.

The Regional Board had not originally contemplated having to provide any ward or beds to take the place of the R.N.H. when it closed; it was, I think, supposed that the few cases of Tuberculosis which still required hospital care might be sent to Portsmouth, and other provision was not necessary.

However statistics revealed that over the decade a significant number of Island patients had been occupying beds there, and that loss of all these beds would leave the service seriously impaired. After several plans had been considered, a new ward to the west of the Upper Hospital and linked to it by a covered corridor was built with 28 beds. This ward was at the time the most modern in the Island hospitals and was built on what was then called the racetrack principle.

It included eight single wards, two double and four 4-bedded, which gave scope for accommodating special groups of patients, - e.g. those with Tuberculosis or other infections. The wards were around the periphery of the building, and bathrooms, storage rooms, clinical rooms - including a small theatre where bronchoscopies and later other endoscopic procedures could be done - were in the centre of the block; these central rooms were lighted by top lights, the corridor roof being about 18 inches lower than the central and peripheral rooms. They had oxygen and suction laid on to each bed. The disadvantage of the plan was that from the nurses' station in the centre of the ward at best only two out of 28 patients could be seen.

This ward was occupied on April 15th 1964 and officially opened by Mark Woodnut, M.P. shortly after this; he named it Hassall Ward commemorating the founder of the R.N.H.

Another separate new ward - Barton Ward - was built at St. Mary's soon after this, to the south of the main hospital, with 30 beds, for men and women, intended for the Geriatric service; it was opened in 1967 by Mrs Barton, a councillor and member of the H.M.C., who had for a long time interested herself in provision for old people; - the Chairman remarking that if there had not been a parish on the Island named Barton we should have had to create one. Before it was occupied it was allocated not to the Geriatric Department but to the Obstetric service, the existing Obstetric ward being in urgent need of upgrading; labour wards and a small operating theatre were provided in the single rooms of Barton Ward and this occupation continued for about a year, - the ward then becoming available for its original purpose, an admission and assessment ward for the Geriatric service.

About this time a small chapel was built just to the east of Barton Ward; it was available for all denominations. This new chapel had two small stained glass windows which had been removed from the chapel of the Royal National Hospital when it was demolished. Like Barton Ward it had a short life. They were both among the first casualties when the new hospital was built.

The next important building at St. Mary's was the Postgraduate Medical Centre. Continuing instruction and education for practising doctors had by now become a well recognised need; opportunity to keep in touch with new practices which develop so much more rapidly now than they did earlier; and every hospital group was now expected to provide a centre where lectures, seminars, tutorials and discussions could take place, and where there would be a good library giving access to a reasonable selection of medical journals and books. Some pioneer work in this line had been done by the Isle of Wight Medical Club which was started in the 1930s by a group of doctors, some G.P.s and some working in hospitals, who met once a month, at first in their own and each other's houses, and later in one or other hospital, to hear someone talk on a subject of interest and to discuss it. Accommodation limited the numbers of doctors who could participate, and the club for several years restricted its membership to 30; but this left out an increasing number and by the end of the 1950s it was agreed that the club must be opened for all doctors practising on the Island; it has to be confessed with regret that lady doctors were for some years excluded, a decision to admit them deferred because a single adverse vote sufficed to defeat the proposition that they should be invited to join!

Some attempts at further meetings had been made earlier; the local branch of the B.M.A. arranged three excellent lectures at intervals, one year in the 1950s, and after the new Out-patient Departments were opened in Ryde and in Newport, Doctor Harland, as Postgraduate Clinical Tutor, arranged a meeting once a month at these hospitals alternately, at which cases were discussed and demonstrated; but it was not until the Postgraduate Medical Centre was opened by Lord Rosenheim, President of the Royal College of Physicians, in October 1966, that the club had a really adequate meeting place, - and its meetings were before long replaced by regular weekly clinical meetings at mid-day on one day of the week, arranged by the clinical tutors, with a speaker, sometimes from the Island staff, often from the mainland, especially from Portsmouth or Southampton. The cost of this new centre was paid in part by the doctors, all the hospital consultants and many General Practitioners contributing. A handsome pastiche 'the Birds' was presented to the centre by the artists who created it - Daisy Krishmanna and Elisabeth Greene: it hung there for about 25 years, before being moved to the new Hospital where it will be seen by more passers-by.

The X-ray Department in the Out-patient building as mentioned was substantially enlarged and modernised and a second consultant appointed; but it was still necessary for all in-patients who required X-ray examination to go down to the Out-patient building, many of them of course had to be taken down by stretcher or in a wheelchair. An accessory X-ray room and equipment was now provided, the room built filling in a gap on the south side of the corridor leading to the theatre and to the two small wards associated with it.

The new kitchens and dining room (or restaurant), built on the north-east side of the hospital and reached by a long corridor from the Upper Hospital, were opened in 1973 and were associated with a new style of delivering meals to the wards. Hitherto, meals had been served on the wards having been taken to them in hot-lock cabinets; there were separate kitchens for Upper and Lower Hospitals and adequate serving kitchens on each ward; once good trolleys were available which would plug in to the mains supply on reaching their destination, it was generally possible for food to be kept properly heated up to the moment of serving. This was the old style. In the new system all meals were served in the kitchen itself and taken on covered plates in trolleys, kept hot, to the wards. Each system has, perhaps, its good points and its less good. Ideally with the old system the ward Sister served each patient; she knew her patients and gave each one what she judged he or she would like, would need, or be able to manage;

the serving of the main meal of the day was often something of a nodal point in the day's programme and a minor but important ceremony; in the Brompton Hospital where I worked as a junior for a year, it was sometimes dubbed by the (often Irish) nurses 'High Mass'. The new system lost all that. Helpings were of standard size when delivered and those who served them saw no more of them, never knowing whether they were consumed or wasted. The trolleys designed for indoor corridors (albeit long ones) found the going difficult up and down the paths leading from the Upper to the Lower Hospitals and round many corners; and at first spillages occurred; and the deliveries took a surprisingly long time so that the meals in different wards had to be staggered over a period of an hour, which was sometimes inconvenient in other ways.

The new kitchens were able to produce and serve meals for the whole hospital, patients, staff and visitors, and the staff dining room became a popular meeting place for meals and a convenient one for informal meetings after post-prandial coffee, etc. Included in new buildings were offices for the catering supervisor and dietitian, stores, changing rooms, etc. This new department, like some others, was to have only a rather short life of no more than about twenty years before it was replaced by the new hospital; it has become in part a linen store and in part serves other purposes.

Further over to the east side of the grounds, a new store was provided; hitherto the hospital stores had been squeezed into the wing which had been previously the hospital chapel; or into the basement; or wherever else room could be found; for example, in the old barn near the back gate onto Dodnor Lane. The new store must have been a great improvement for the engineering, building and maintenance departments and it also provided good accommodation for the central sterile supplies; a new telephone exchange was provided adjacent to the store, - moved from the porter's lodge where it had been since 1949.

On the north side of the open square, formed by the new dining room and kitchen block on the west and the stores on the east, was the new Pathology laboratory. Up until nearly this time one Consultant Pathologist had worked alone on the Island with his staff; the department was, as it always had been, associated with the Pathology service in Portsmouth, and some of the routine work was done there; also, as mentioned, a small department functioned in the Royal National Hospital up to the time of its closure; and visiting technicians held clinics in Shanklin at the Arthur Webster Institute and in East Cowes at the Frank James Hospital; but most of the work was done at Ryde or at St. Mary's. Now the new department was intended to provide adequate accommodation for all types of Pathology at St. Mary's; but the laboratory at

Ryde remained open and, so long as a large proportion of both in-patient and out-patient remained there, work continued at Ryde as there was obvious need for it; moreover the new department at St. Mary's had soon to be enlarged by the addition of Portakabins.

Resident medical staff had increased in numbers and, for the registrars, three small houses were built, - the first by the then main entrance, - Apple Gate, - and two later ones off Dodnor Lane, Almond-Gate and Cherry-Gate. New nurses' homes had been built, but it was the custom among nurses at the time to live out rather than in; consequently there was accommodation to spare and the upper floor of the old nurses' quarters, in the middle of the main hospital, was for a time converted into quarters for a Houseman.

When the relief road for Newport/Cowes was built, the hospital had to surrender a large corner of its ground, as already mentioned; the cricket field had from 1950 onwards been used as a helicopter landing pad; the hospital was in fact the first in the country to make use of the helicopter service; later after this field was reduced in size helicopters landed on the sloping field below the nurses' home, where just now a new landing pad has been marked out. A further part of the cricket field was taken about 1978 for the building of the Geriatric Day Hospital.

Another new building was the hospital Social Club which since then has remained a popular and much used centre for social activities for the staff.

With all the new building, the human side was not forgotten; visiting hours in the early days had been extremely limited: so late as 1949, for example, visiting in the childrens' ward (at Ryde) had been limited to one hour a week on Sundays, for parents only,

Now in 1968, the committee decided on unrestricted visiting in all wards, with some limitations in childrens' and surgical wards.

Sadly, this led to unanticipated difficulties: some relations and friends mistakenly thought that they would only show proper concern by remaining by the patient's bedside, or chairside, for long hours; that their anxiety for the patient's progress would be deemed commensurate with the length of their stay: and some, it must be said, were prepared to use the ward's day-room as a vicarious television lounge. After a few months, visiting had to be limited to 5.00 p.m. - 8.00 p.m. or 2.00 p.m. - 8.00 p.m. on Sundays, with sisters being given discretion to impose restrictions locally.

At the start of the N.H.S. Whitecroft was acknowledged to be overcrowded; this remained the case and was attributed especially to the large number of elderly patients, and in 1953 there was consideration of building an annexe for 76 beds to house some of these patients, and also of a 'Mental Deficiency Unit' of 84 patients; it was first suggested that this should be in a ten acre area (Hungry Hill) within the grounds of Whitecroft; it was also proposed at one time to purchase Gatcombe House as a convalescent home for mental patients: neither of these schemes went any further.

The annual report in 1955 mentioned that of 271 admissions during that year, 73.8% were voluntary; there were 42 deaths, of which 36 were in patients over 65. The report refers to Out-patient clinics at Ryde, St. Mary's, Frank James and Whitecroft and to E.C.T. Out-patient clinics at Whitecroft; also to domiciliary visits.

The next year, Longford Sanatorium became available and a transfer of women and girls from St. Mary's was soon arranged; the commissioners of the Board of Control, reporting that year, approved the use of the Catherine Bowen Home for 16 girls; they commented on the shortage of nursing staff at Whitecroft, - a national problem - where there were then 37 male and 26 female nurses plus 10 part-time women, 9 students and 8 ward orderlies at night; they gave a favourable report upon the amenities and general management of the hospital; later that year the annual report for Whitecroft mentions the hope of converting farm buildings into geriatric accommodation. It was in this year that an additional consultant was appointed at Whitecroft. The building of a 'mental colony' off Dodnor Lane close to St. Mary's had been another of the earliest projects considered by the H.M.C. though obviously it never came to fruition; another plan was the establishment of a central laundry at Whitecroft which did come about.

A rather different, unexpected, question arose in 1957, namely the legality of patients at Whitecroft serving as beaters; presumably local shooting parties patronised by or joined by the staff needed such assistance; the opinion of the Board's Legal Adviser was sought, and was non-committal!

Throughout this phase, as before, many residents at Whitecroft and in the mentally defective wards at St. Mary's worked in the hospitals. Four-fifths of the patients in Whitwell Ward in St. Mary's did work of some sort there, receiving five shillings weekly plus a half to one ounce of tobacco or cigarettes or sweets. Men worked in the gardens or on the farms while they existed; and women worked in the laundry or in the hospital.

In July 1958 a particularly troublesome strain of Staphylococcus aureus ('phage 80) was causing concern at Whitecroft; it was deemed advisable to empty one large ward so it could be cleaned and fumigated; 45 patients were transferred to the Royal National Hospital and a few others to Fairlee and others were housed temporarily in the large hall at Whitecroft.

In March 1959 Thompson House was opened, taking patients back from the R.N.H. and a number from St. Mary's; named after the late Alderman Thompson who had been associated with Whitecroft for 38 years. The wards at Whitecroft had been given names, - the Medical Superintendent was invited to choose the names and had selected national poets and explorers; in 1960 reception wards were created partly by the change of use for the Superintendent's quarters; the training schools and occupational therapy departments were improved and in 1963 a chapel was dedicated. The two new wards in Thompson House were given the up-to-date names of Neil Armstrong and T.S. Eliot.

By 1968 the closure of Whitecroft was in the air, - a working party advised the building of a mental health centre and short stay beds at St. Mary's, - not to await the building of the district hospital; and in the following year some progress was made in transferring elderly patients from the hospital to residential homes. Old fashioned treatments were being abandoned; four padded rooms were abolished, - one remained but unlocked; and new forms of treatment were being adopted which would themselves in time become outdated. An anaesthetist visited regularly for a time to assist at electro-convulsion treatment, and for at least two years Mr. Wylie McCissock from the Atkinson-Morley Hospital visited to carry out Frontal Leucotomy for a few patients; for this purpose the theatre at St. Mary's was used. In 1971 the position of Medical Superintendent was abandoned, Doctor McBryde who had replaced Doctor Gordon-Brown in 1966 remained as one of three consultants; the next year the psychiatrists decided they could give the best service if the Island were divided into three sectors, each consultant accepting responsibility for one sector. The Island like all Gaul was duly quartered into three halves and the arrangement continues at the present.

Throughout the Health Service, the rule was that hospital beds were allocated to consultants who had the right and obligation to admit and discharge patients; every patient must be, at least nominally, under the care of a consultant, who must accept responsibility; this was straightforward enough in general hospitals; in the Cottage Hospitals such as Frank James it necessitated a certain change in style. The General Practitioners however continued to staff the hospital as they had before and to share the on-call duties; if they wished to admit one of their own patients, this had to be done by agreement with the appropriate consultant whose name appeared on their notes; alternatively patients from the locality who found themselves in one of the general hospitals might be transferred, given a vacancy, to the Cottage Hospital, and there attended by their own doctor, while nominally under the care of the consultant who admitted them in the first place.

In fact the paucity of operating theatres in the group led to the Frank James very soon being used in part to supplement the surgical accommodation; regular operating lists were done there in E.N.T. work as already mentioned, by Dr Crosskey in the first place; in general surgery, in Orthopaedic surgery, and in Gynaecology; and inevitably a good deal of ward space was taken up by these patients and the number of beds available for local patients admitted, at the request of the local doctors, diminished. In 1964 a childrens' ward, which I think was, sometimes at least, referred to as Carnt Ward, in recognition of the many services and contributions made by Mr. E.G. Carnt, was taken over as a Gynaecological ward.

Nurses and domestic staff had originally been resident with rooms on the upper floor; by the 1970s, there as elsewhere, most nurses and domestics lived out and space was available for other purposes. A psychotherapy unit was opened in 1972, using part of the upper floor and conducted by Dr Ian Thomson for several years.

To complete the story of the Frank James, in October 1976, the hospital was temporarily closed for refurbishment and re-opened in March 1977 when a decision was made that casualty facilities should no longer be available, and in 1988, as the N.H.S. prepared for further economies, and as the imminent opening of the new St. Mary's called for review of the Health Authority's institutions, that Frank James Hospital should be kept open and should be developed as a community hospital; and this was further considered in a consultancy document in 1990. The mens' ward, in particular, was remodelled to give a number of small wards.

Then in 1992 Geriatric patients from T.S. Eliot Ward which was closed were transferred to the Frank James Hospital.

Recently the building formerly used as a mortuary has been converted into a small chapel available for all creeds and denominations; and the two small stained glass windows which were originally in the chapel of the Royal National Hospital and later moved to the short-lived chapel at St. Mary's have now been installed there.

## Shanklin Hospitals

Shanklin Cottage Hospital, like the Frank James, besides providing some beds for the local population continued to play an important part in the surgical services for the whole Island. A wing had been built providing eight private or amenity beds; besides these there were six beds kept for children, - usually a weekly list of tonsillectomies; and eight or nine others for medical or surgical patients; surgery included general surgical, orthopaedic and gynaecological lists, done generally by one of the General Practitioners with qualifications and experience. The small wards were re-decorated and re-arranged and a small glass fronted day room was provided.

As the years went on there was much concern and discussion about the future use of the hospital; the demand throughout this time was especially for beds for the elderly sick, and the feeling was that when medical cases were admitted they usually came in that category, and that such patients were unlikely to be discharged unless after a long wait they were transferred to the Geriatric Wards; consequently there was a very small turnover of patients. The declared intention was to retain the hospital as a local community or General Practitioner hospital; lack of adequate funds made it impossible to fulfil this plan, and the hospital was closed with the intention, or at least the hope, of re-opening it in time; but sadly a fire seems to have put an end to this hope.

At the Arthur Webster Institute sessions were held on five days a week for physiotherapy, and an orthopaedic surgeon attended twice weekly. A consultant in psychology held one clinic a week and the psychiatric social worker attended there on three evenings and a speech therapist once a week. And there was a dental surgery there and a social club for patients; finally the buildings provide a garage for the Ambulance Service; there was a caretaker's flat until 1982 when as part of an 'economy drive' it was felt that a caretaker was no longer necessary.

XIV

# THE HEALTH AUTHORITIES

The final meeting of the H.M.C. was early in 1974 and the initial meeting of the Area Health Authority in March that year; the Chairman, Mrs. Thelma Margham and the Vice Chairman, Admiral J.L. Blackham and several other members of the Authority had been members of the H.M.C., which was now abolished and replaced by Area and District Health Authorities; and the administration of the Public Health Department, - Medical, Nursing, Midwifery, Health Visiting, and Ancillary Departments, shifted from the Local Authority to the Health Authorities. The Regional Authorities remained.

It was originally intended that the Island should be managed by a District Authority which would be subordinate to an Area Health Authority, that would include Portsmouth and Southampton; it was, however, believed on the Island that no matter how fair the intentions of the managing bodies, our rural population of about 120,000 would have very little say and very low priority with the two massive populations on the other side of the Solent; representations had been made however, for the independence of the Island and were, much to the relief of the Island Authorities, accepted; and the Island H.A. remained on its own and answerable to the region, not becoming what must have been a very small component of a very large authority across the water. Possibly the successful campaign for the Island to remain a separate county, eagerly desired and enthusiastically celebrated at County Hall, was one factor in the decision, since one objective of the new administration was that Area Health and Local Government authorities should be co-terminous.

The years of 1974 to 1992 were a time of increase in all directions; there were more nurses, though all too often not nearly enough, more doctors, senior and junior, (lots) more administrators, more money and more buildings; with the rising population more patients and especially more elderly patients; more clinics, more physiotherapists, occupational therapists, speech therapists, chiropodists, radiographers, laboratory scientists, pharmacists, secretaries, clerks, accountants, - where does the list end? There were perhaps no more gardeners, no more cooks and no more porters, without the intention of belittling in the smallest way the important service of these categories.

At the outset Francis Eade retired and Mr. J. Parker became the Area

Administrator; G.F. Hardy continued as treasurer; Doctor F. Ellis Henderson was appointed Community Physician and Doctor R.K. Machell, the County Medical Officer left for another appointment; Miss Pilbeam was the Principal Nursing Officer, Mr. Tombs the Personnel Officer; these five with representatives of the Consultants (A.B. Oliveira) and the General Practitioners (J.G. Sandiford) and their deputies made up the Area Management team, which met monthly and reported to the Area Health Authority. They could co-opt others if necessary, for example Mr. W. Maden, the Area Dental Officer.

The A.H.A. continued with some changes in personnel until 1982; then in another re-organisation, Area Authorities were eliminated, the Island became a District with relatively slight changes, save in the titles of the officers, etc. It was, however, at this juncture that Mrs. Margham retired and the Chairmanship passed to Group Captain Naylor who continued until 1988, when, to the expressed regret of his committee, he was not re-appointed; his place was filled by Mr. C.G.J. Bland, and after another two years by Major-General Brian Livesey, who presided over the last years of the D.H.A. and the first few of the new Isle of Wight Health Commission. The new District Authority after 1982 was known simply as the Isle of Wight Health Authority.

The new St. Mary's was planned and building began in 1983. The acquisition of a coat of arms was considered, and enquiries made to the College of Heralds as to the cost; and in due course suitable arms were provided for the I.o.W. Health Authority. Mr. Parker retired and Mr. A. Blee became the Administrator and in 1985 the District General Manager; and Mr. M. Powell became the Chief Administrator at St. Mary's.

The King Edward Foundation pointed out that a number of necessary services could not be available in the new hospital as planned; the plans would leave a need for an additional medical ward, a department of Ophthalmology and for Rheumatology and Rehabilitation and they might have added for Dentistry or Orofacial surgery and for Physiotherapy; and provision would be needed for mental illness and for the mentally handicapped and for the group classified as Elderly Severely Mentally Ill (E.S.M.I.); it was reckoned that a 60-bedded unit for mental illness would be needed as well as 98 beds for the class of E.S.M.I. currently accommodated at Whitecroft; and many suggestions as to their accommodation were made; also for the 96 mentally handicapped presently at Whitecroft; there was already a provision for 25 children at Castleview; the use of one or more wards at Ryde or Shanklin or the creation of group homes were all considered.

Changes in management were made at this time, the work of the hospitals being divided into the Acute Services; maternity, child health and primary care;

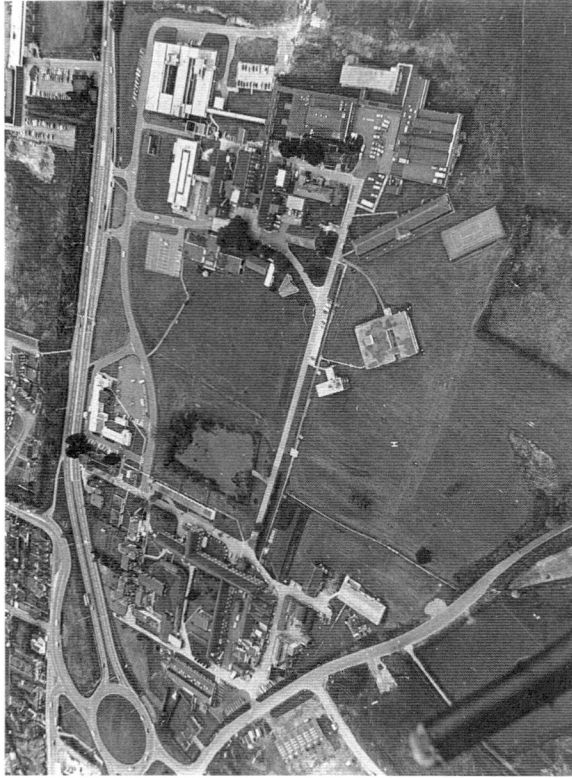

**Plate 14**. An aerial view of St. Mary's Hospital about 1980. The sloping field between the pond and the buildings of the Upper (north) Hospital became the site of the new hospital. Top left is the Obstetric wing and below that Hassall Ward (now the Mottistone wing), further down is the old Out-patient & X-ray department and, by the trees, the porter's lodge, offices and the former main entrance.

Near the round-about are two doctors' houses and the Geriatric Day Hospital and the entrance from Dodnor Lane: further up this lane is the Ambulance station, - the new entrance from the lane has not yet been constructed. To the right of the drive between Upper & Lower Hospital are the two nurses' homes and the nurse training school. On the left the chapel and Barton Ward are separated by some temporary buildings. At the top are the Stores, the Pathology Laboratory and the new kitchens and dining-rooms. Compared with all this, the buildings of the old Infirmary look very small! Newcroft Hospital and Margham House are yet to come. *Courtesy: Pam Osborne.*

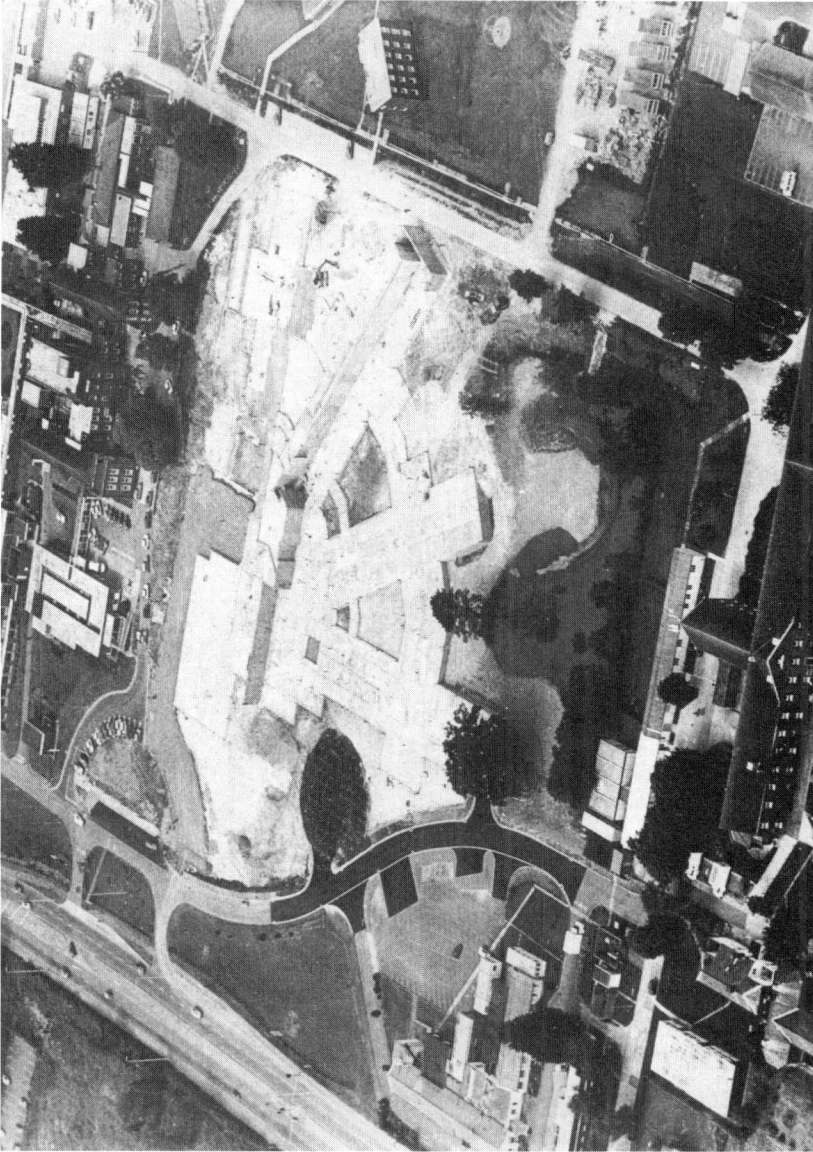

**Plate 15.** The shape of things to come - the new hospital under construction. Barton Ward and the Chapel have been demolished. *Courtesy: Mr. J. Lewis (& others?).*

179

mental illness; mental handicap; and the elderly. Each service would have and manage its own budget; and there were also to be Management Authorities for administration, for records, which now became 'Patient Services', catering, engineering, building, energy and estate management and miscellaneous departments; there were also the District Services to be considered - Pathology, Pharmacy, Personnel and Planning, Dentistry, Psychology, Catering, Domestics, Works and Supplies. With a new hospital looming up, the future of Ryde Hospital and the Casualty Department had to be considered. At this stage the local medical committee, the General Practitioners Committee, in 1982 thought it should be kept open. The available beds for the elderly, based upon the number of elderly in the community, were a long way below the national average. It was at this time suggested that General Practitioner beds, i.e. beds into which General Practitioners could admit and care for their own patients, should be retained at Frank James Hospital and at Shanklin and Ryde Hospitals.

A preliminary measure to the building of the new hospital was the demolition of Barton Ward after a mere 18 years of life; and also of the small chapel near it. Some temporary rooms for community nurses had been set up under the trees between the main hospital and Barton Ward and these too had to go. Barton Ward was moved, name and all, to the pre-fabricated buildings which had been the up-graded Whitwell Ward for mentally handicapped boys and men, holding 37 patients who were now transferred to Whitecroft. 24 'low dependency' patients remained in Seaview Villa in the Lower Hospital.


In 1964 about the time of the closure of the Royal National Hospital there were 16 consultants working on the Island and a number of visiting consultants coming from Portsmouth or Southampton or elsewhere for sessions weekly or less often. 25 years later the number of consultants increased to about 35 and new departments have been opened dealing with Paediatrics, Geriatrics, Dermatology, Rheumatology, Genito-urinary medicine, Dental surgery, Child psychology; Neurology, Cardiology and Plastic surgery are still provided for by visiting consultants. At the same time of course junior staff have greatly increased. In 1964 at St. Mary's there was one house physician who was required to cover the whole of general medicine and the geriatric wards, one house surgeon, one casualty house surgeon and one obstetric house surgeon. At that time there was only one registrar working on the Island, a medical registrar who had previously divided his time between Ryde and the Royal National Hospital; now with that closed he worked at Newport and Ryde. Increase in the resident medical staff at St. Mary's called for new accommodation and a new building to the east of the other hospital buildings was to be put up, now providing accommodation for five medical residents. It also allowed a trial in style and building technique preliminary to the new hospital; it was named Margham House in recognition of Mrs. Margham's services to the H.M.C. and the A.H.A. over the years.

At the start of the A.H.A.'s term of office the total nursing establishment on the Island was 769, - of which 698 worked in hospitals and 71 in the community. There were 1040 beds, all but five available for use, and an average bed occupancy of about 80%. In the first year 2753 patients were discharged or died.

At this time too, the non-medical and non-nursing staff employed by the Authority included 8 electricians, 1 general foreman, 8 fitters and plumbers, 6 labourers, 7 carpenters, 6 painters and 5 bricklayers; there were 10 area administrators and their assistants; and there were also 12 chaplains of all denominations giving services in the 7 hospitals. The central pharmacy for the group had been established by the H.M.C. years earlier; it remained throughout these years in the pre-fabricated building to the north of the main drive; in 1979 the pharmacy staff numbered 10, it was thought then that there should be two or three more.

The Ambulance Service, hitherto administered by the County, now also passed to the A.H.A.; the service had shared accommodation and to some degree management with the Fire Service; but this now came to an end and a building in Carisbrooke Road had to be leased temporarily, until a new Ambulance Station was built at St. Mary's with the entrance off Dodnor Lane. When the Ambulance Service was taken over there were 12 ambulances on the Island. The introduction of a geriatric day hospital in 1978 substantially increased the load on the Ambulance Service. Ambulances continued to be stationed at Ryde, Shanklin, Freshwater and Cowes.

The headquarters of the H.M.C. had been at Whitecroft and these were taken over by the A.H.A., and an additional building, described as temporary, was set up to accommodate the administrative staff; 20 years later it is still in full use.

The new Authority, in one of its earliest meetings, had deplored the building of an industrial estate on the opposite side of Dodnor Lane; believing that it would be disturbingly close to a development for mentally handicapped patients which at that time was intended in the north east part of the grounds; but this of course never came about, although the industrial estate did.

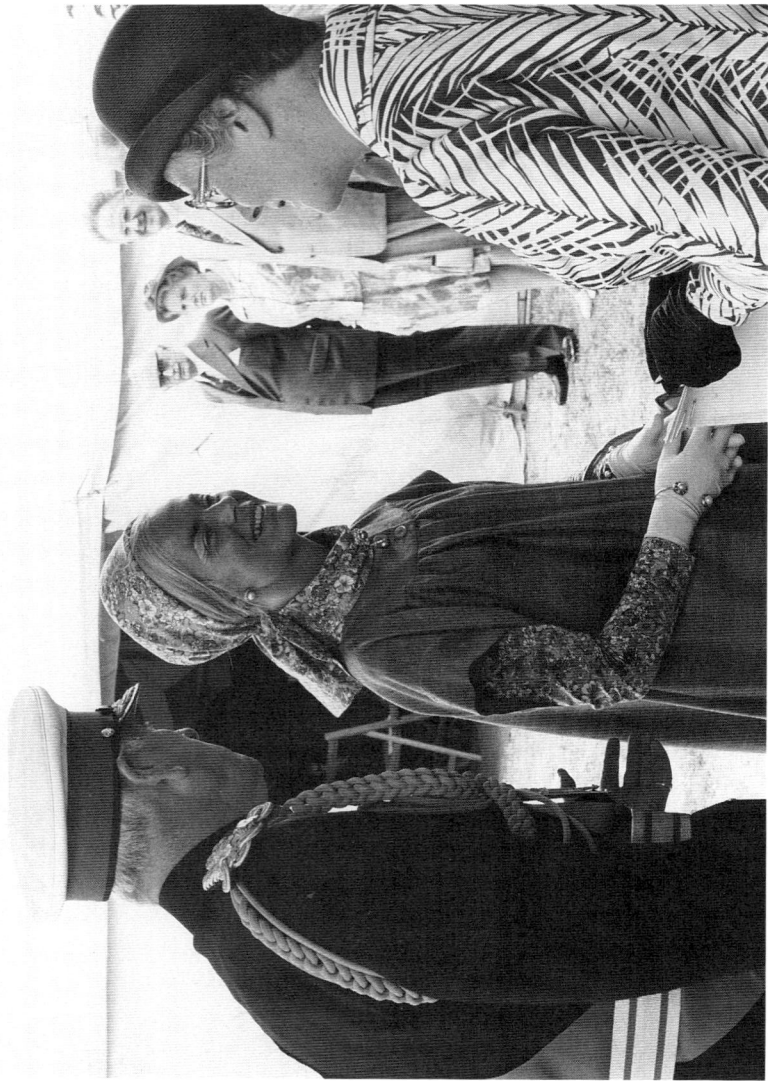

**Plate 16.** The Duchess of Kent with Mrs. Thelma Margham at the opening of the Obstetric wing, 1976 (Also in the picture are Earl Mountbatten, Mr. G. R. Hardy & Dr Ellis Henderson). *Courtesy: Mrs. T. Margham.*

The building of the new Obstetric Unit had been planned and set in train before the changes of administration, and the sound of pile-driving became all too familiar to those who worked in, or who were temporarily warded in, the Upper Hospital or Hassall Ward, - as indeed it did a decade later when the new St. Mary's was going up. The building which was never given a particular name, although the wards were named Osborne and Freshwater after the wards in the old St. Mary's previously used for obstetrics, was opened on July 15th, 1976, by the Duchess of Kent; and now at last the Island had a department which gave excellent accommodation for all aspects of obstetrics; for the mothers, the infants, nurses and midwives, Obstetricians, ante-natal clinics, neonatal care. Mr. and Mrs. W. Edwards who had had much to do with planning the building, had by then left the hospital, but were invited back for the occasion. It was the Chairman's particular desire to have a really first class department and it must have been with very great pleasure that she greeted the Duchess of Kent on that occasion. The Duchess did an un-hurried walk-about after the opening ceremony, meeting many staff and patients, and wrote subsequently recording her thanks to the members and staff of the Authority for an extremely happy occasion.

The opening of this new department liberated the ground floor wards, hitherto used for obstetrics, and there was I think never much doubt about the use to which they must be put, although the claims of the department of Rheumatology and Re-habilitation were considered also; but the long awaited paediatric wards were at last established there after considerable re-building and re-modelling; and the new wards were still not entirely freed of the incubus of the corridor from surgical wards to the theatre; it was still a few years before this department was opened but, once available, it provided, I believe, a considerable improvement in the hospital service with the Paediatric staff, both senior and junior, able to work when necessary in close association with the Obstetric wards and neonatal nurseries. The rooms on the south side of the ground floor of the central block which had seen so many different uses, now became the Paediatrician's headquarters with his secretary's office etc. there.

There were changes in the Lower Hospital during these years. Day room accommodation in the two ladies' geriatric wards, Rookwood and Newport, had been altogether absent when the Geriatric Department was first set up in 1961; they had been up-graded about the time that Barton Ward had been built, and some attempts had been made to provide day rooms; but with the space available they were inevitably poor and crowded and, one must say, miserably inadequate. Large day rooms were built now for these two wards in the 1970s and a lift installed, a great improvement; and in the 1980s both wards in turn were once more up-graded, providing after much effort two acceptable modern wards. Newport became one of the principal medical wards for St. Mary's and despite the building of the new hospital still fulfils that function. In the changing scene this involved a loss of beds for the Geriatric Department.

A Geriatric day hospital was built and opened in 1978. After much planning and discussion a standard design, used in several other places in the region, was accepted and was built on the south side of the Lower Hospital with an entrance from Dodnor Lane. This has provided scope for Geriatric day patients, for their physiotherapy, occupational therapy and re-habilitation and training; and its facilities have been shared to a degree with the Department of Rheumatology and Re-habilitation, and out of hospital hours have provided a location for a stroke club. The men's ward in the Lower Hospital, St. Catherine's, which from the start of the Geriatric Unit was run on two floors was also substantially up-graded in the early 1980s with a new day room built on the north side facing the main drive; this has now become the Re-habilitation ward; the upstairs section which already had reasonably spacious day accommodation remained a long-stay ward for men for some time but that, too, has now been taken over for other purposes.

Of the two separate buildings on the west side one, before Barton Ward was built, had been the ladies admission ward for the Geriatric service and later had served as a re-habilitation ward; the other continued to house some of the mentally handicapped men and boys; the former, known as Holly House and formerly as Wootton Ward, has been considerably modified and has now come to provide offices for the Occupational Health Service and for Personnel Departments; the other, formerly Seaview Villa, also much altered, has become the Diabetic Centre, conceived and managed by Dr Arun Baksi. The third building in that line, once the Chaplain's and then the Master's house has since 1948 been used as offices and continues that function now.

In the Upper Hospital two small wards were separated from the main medical ward for coronary care or later intensive care; and similar provision of one single ward was made in the County Hospital in Harington Ward. There, also, a day room was built on at the east front of Cottle Ward.

The move of the Paediatric Wards to St. Mary's freed Victoria Ward, in Ryde, for other purposes; for some time it was used to accommodate patients moved from other wards in the hospital while these were being redecorated and later some orthopaedic beds were provided there; but it became, for a time, the in-patient accommodation for the Department of Rheumatology and Re-habilitation. However, when in 1985 it was decided to move all medical beds to St. Mary's the Rheumatology department, more concerned with day patients and out-patients, kept its headquarters in Partlands Avenue in the Department of Physiotherapy and has also shared the Geriatric day hospital.

The introduction of hip surgery called for improvements in the theatre at Newport and it was not appropriate for Dental Surgery to use the same theatre; in 1979 a new Dental Clinic was opened at St. Mary's occupying rooms associated in the early days of the hospital with its first midwifery department. In later years the remaining and larger part of this block was turned into a theatre with its ancillary rooms and recovery room for day surgery. The main theatre was up-graded, the small adjacent ward, Bonchurch Ward, was used for orthopaedic surgery. At Ryde the operating theatre and associated rooms were up-graded in 1981/1982; but earlier than this in the 1970s the Casualty Department, now more correctly known as the Accident and Emergency Centre, was re-modelled again and two small theatres were made available there; and it remained the principal 'A and E' Department until 1992; at Newport the Casualty Department had sometimes, for lack of staff, again to be closed, or its operation limited to 9 a.m. to 5 p.m. on five days weekly. It had become partly dependent upon the work of retired practitioners, - and particularly, latterly, Doctor O'Meara, - for its medical staff, and when he finally retired it seemed for a time that it would have to be closed.

An early obligation of the A.H.A. was to assume managerial control of the pathology services, which up until then had been part of the Portsmouth and Isle of Wight service. With only one consultant resident on the Island this would not be achieved at once, and very soon there were plans to increase the numbers of consultants; at first a consultant worked here part time dividing his sessions between the Island and Portsmouth; but soon there was first one, then two and then three additional consultants residing on the Island and working full time there. The laboratory at Ryde continued in use, but the new department at St. Mary's became the headquarters of Haematology, Microbiology and Biochemistry, and large though it seemed in comparison with the earlier laboratory, it was soon found to be in need of expansion; and in 1979 two Portakabins were provided to give additional space for laboratory, storage, and waiting rooms; among other things the advent of anti-coagulant management had added very considerably to the load. A further Portakabin was needed in 1982 to give more room for biochemical work.

As the scope of pathology increased and the number of investigations rose exponentially, difficulties developed over out-of-hours calls. With the relatively small Island population, each sub-division of the Pathology Department could only have a few, - perhaps one or two - trained technicians working in that particular discipline; but each would not necessarily be able to carry out all the emergency investigations sought in other sub-specialities; moreover, up to about 1970 technicians had generally agreed to attend the hospital, if called out, regarding this as a purely voluntary concession; the increasing numbers of such calls made this no longer a reasonable expectation, and of course was it not feasible to send such emergency demands off the Island. Eventually a satisfactory agreement was reached with limitation in the types of investigation which could properly be regarded as needed in emergencies.

The Central Sterile Supply Department installed after 1974 more or less adjacent to the Pathology building, continued to draw its stock from Portsmouth, and Miss McKay remained the Liaison Officer; she retired in 1982 but continued after that for a while to work part time.


Whitecroft Hospital in 1975 besides providing psychiatric service and accommodation for the administration, also housed the central laundry for the whole group. The group laundry had in fact been there for many years and when Longford Hospital was first used for mentally defective girls and women in 1955 a number of them used to be driven daily to Whitecroft to work in the laundry there. This practice ceased, however, in 1959, and in 1976 the occupational therapy work going on at Longford Hospital was especially commended, and the Authority planned to 're-vamp' (to quote the actual word used in the minutes) the Catherine Bowen Home as an occupational therapy and general training unit. O.T. was an important feature of the daily routine of many patients at Whitecroft and by 1978 trained therapists were working there for some 69 hours a week with untrained assistants for about 164 hours.

The hospital accommodation for aged and demented patients, - the group sometimes known as the Elderly Severely Mentally Ill (E.S.M.I.) or now more commonly known as Alzheimer's Disease, had been a problem both for the Geriatric Department and the psychiatrists, which had mounted in proportion to the increasing number of old people on the Island. In the early years of the service, - and indeed before, - large numbers of them had been admitted to Whitecroft. When the Geriatric Department came into existence, - a dozen years after the N.H.S. began, - it was natural and proper that the psychiatrists should expect some easing of the load.

Over the next few years an amicable agreement was reached between the two departments, roughly that when old people became in need of hospital care, those with some physical disorder, such as a stroke, Parkinson's Disease, or a fractured limb, would appropriately be placed in the Geriatric Wards; when the disability was solely a mental failure, they should be cared for by the psychiatrists. A high proportion of such patients however reached the hospital by way of the A and E department, and had to wait on the medical or surgical wards for a vacancy; vacancies in the Geriatric Wards were usually few since they depended upon a discharge of resident patients; very many of these could only go to the County Council (Part Three) Homes; again an agreement was reached between the hospital side and the social workers as to the proper place for individuals; but since the Geriatric Wards on the one hand and the County Council Homes on the other were both substantially under-provided with the requisite number of beds (i.e. the number recommended for a given population of elderly by the Ministry of Health) both were inevitably and continuously under stress and always unable to do as much as was needed and as they would have wished; furthermore the continuous, and at times almost complete, shortfall in physiotherapy and occupational therapy on the Geriatric Wards for the first 15 to 20 years of their existence compounded the problem.

About the time of the establishment of the A.H.A., 14 beds in Thompson House at Whitecroft were allocated to the Geriatric Department and later after some work on the ward, these were increased to 29. This ward remained part of the Geriatric Department until the closure of the hospital when the patients were transferred to the Frank James Hospital in 1992.

In 1979 the bed complement at Whitecroft was still above 300 although only 248 beds were actually staffed and occupied. 130 patients had been discharged or had died in the previous year, and there had been 1724 attendances by day patients. The psychotherapeutic unit had been active at Frank James Hospital, for several years and other such units were also now available.

Along with the new St. Mary's a new hospital 'Newcroft' for mental illnesses was built, on land within the original allocation of 80 acres of Parkhurst Forest made over to the guardians more than 200 years ago. The Guardians had turned down the County Council's suggestion of building a mental hospital there about 1890, and it must be that the land now used was more or less what had been refused a century earlier. The contrast between Newcroft Hospital in 1992 and Whitecroft Hospital in 1948 is very great; it should be understood that Whitecroft in its day was considered, for example by the Commissioners in Lunacy, and the Inspectors from the Ministry of Health later, to be a good mental hospital, up-to-date with patients well cared for and with good occupational therapy. The contrast must be attributed to changes in ideas and management. Fifty years ago Whitecroft, with almost ten times the number of beds that there are now at Newcroft, and serving a population about 25% smaller than now, was overcrowded. Now besides Newcroft there are a number of psychotherapy centres, and houses for elderly patients classified as suffering from Alzheimer's Disease; and several centres where community services, social services, etc., co-operate with the psychiatrists; and of course there are a great many private residential and nursing homes. It is in such centres and homes that many of those who would have been patients in Whitecroft, or St. Mary's, in years gone by must now, with the help of their General Practitioners, be treated and managed. How successful and effective these changes are is, one is glad to say, a matter outside the scope of this book.

A feature of the new administration was the creation of Community Health Councils; each Authority included such a Council with members, 18 on the Island, appointed by Local Authorities, by the Regional Health Authority, and as to one third of them, by the local charitable organisations; these numerous organisations balloted among themselves for their representatives. The function of these Councils was, and is, to be a link between the people, i.e. the local population, and the Authority; they have been termed 'Consumer's Watchdog'; they have the rights to be consulted on major strategic developments in the area; to visit hospitals and any other properties of the Authority, e.g. clinics; and to receive and consider complaints relating both to the hospital and to general practice; they meet monthly and are entitled to send an observer to all area or district meetings for which an agenda is published. On the Island they consider, among other matters, such things as access for the disabled to hospital buildings, clinics, etc; and they have issued guides and information pamphlets. The first Chairman was Douglas Gordon a former Mayor of Newport and Chairman of B.L.E.S.M.A., with Archdeacon Scruby his Vice-Chairman.

Many voluntary services have played perhaps an increasing part in the life and activities of the hospitals although they were not, most of them, new. The Guild of Past Patients at the Royal County Hospital was founded early in the 1950s and the League of Friends of St. Mary's had become a wide ranging business-like activity and a registered charity before the present phase. Among other things it now runs the hospital shop and cafeteria and had made many important gifts to the hospital, - the greatest one, which involved the energies of many members over years, being the Body Scanner, the accumulated funds for which amounted to nearly three-quarters of a million pounds; another item of major importance is the Endoscope Appeal Fund; but it must not be thought that gifts were limited to certain major items alone; they included such things as help towards the Coronary Care Unit at Ryde in 1971 and the day rooms in 1978 and the provision of two special baths, E.N.T. equipment, a hoist, stethoscope headphones and many other things. Their income is derived from subscriptions, donations, street collections and sales in shops and cafeteria; when Ryde Hospital closed the Guild of Past Patients joined the Friends of St. Mary's and brought with them assets of £10,000.

The W.R.V.S. managed and manned the canteens for Out Patients at Ryde and Newport, the latter jointly with Toc H, the Baptist Church, the Red Cross, and the Inner Wheel. Library services are of great value and I believe importance, to the patients; the library service for the Island was provided through a joint committee of the Red Cross and St. John's Ambulance, - with some contributions from the Friends of the hospital and Toc H. In 1962 Mrs. Ramsden, the County Organiser for the service, mentioned in her report that in all there were then 15 helping in the library service in one hospital or another; 7 of these had had some training in the headquarters of the (National) service; £43 had been available that year for new books and 56 new books had been purchased and 2 automatic page turners, - most valuable items for patients who are unable to use their hands. The library headquarters moved from Ryde to St. Mary's in 1964, and for a time part of the small building just outside the door into St. Catherine's ward was used for a central library. The Red Cross and St. John's also manage the picture library, and provide a trolley shop service for the wards; (sale of tobacco and cigarettes is banned).

The Voluntary Car Service has been operating since the beginning of the Health Service and indeed before that; at first entirely independent, it came to be controlled and organised by the Ambulance Service, - but of course drivers continued to give of their time and their skill, and the service has been much in demand. In 1975, however, while the Ambulance Service was in dispute with the management of the N.H.S. it was suspended for a few weeks except for emergency work. In May 1984 the D.H.A. paid a tribute to the service of the voluntary car drivers and a presentation was made to two senior drivers whose services had been outstanding.

Besides these various activities, actual voluntary work in the hospital under the direction of Sisters and others was undertaken for several years; the service was introduced in 1970 and the first report was considered rather disappointing; later Mr. Scotcher was appointed head of this service and was able to produce effective and useful results. This was a time when management and staff were more than usually concerned at the stress laid upon the nursing and also upon the portering and domestic staff, simply by the volume of work required. The use of voluntary workers aimed at relieving this stress by arranging for some jobs to be done by volunteers. The cynical may say that it was a scheme whereby some of the necessary work was done free of charge; alternatively it could be claimed that it was a useful way of harnessing the good will of the community and putting it to use to improve the service while encouraging the local population to feel that they were contributing to the effectiveness and value of their hospital. By 1975 Mr. Scotcher had a roll of 437 volunteers who had offered their services in one way or another. Many hours of work were booked for each week; work included transport for relatives to or from hospital; escorts to clinics or between hospitals; help with the hospital receptions; transport during ambulance disputes; and during an epidemic of flu, when many staff were off sick, help with actual nursing.

Apart from all this the writer can recall with gratitude a number of people who quite independently of any particular organisation regularly visited seriously disabled patients simply to talk to them, read to them, or just keep them company for a while; such visits are of very real value.

This does not complete the list. Many other organisations have made their contributions over the years - the Lions, the Rotarians, the Inner Wheel, the Buccaneers who provided the verandah for Barton Ward, the Townswomen's Guild, the Women's Institutes, Churches and Chapels, the Carnival Committees and others including many individuals who have made substantial bequests or donations.


At the Post Graduate Medical Centre, opened in 1966, Doctor Harland, the first clinical tutor was followed by Doctor Philip James, Doctor David Hide and Doctor Alan Logan. The medical centre and tutors and, indeed, all senior medical staff became affiliated to the Southampton Medical School, and some medical students from Southampton spend some of their time of clinical instruction at St. Mary's. Clinical meetings were held at first in the evenings but more recently there have been regular mid-week lunch hour meetings with talks by resident or visiting consultants and others.

Courses of lectures are given and during the 1980s refresher courses lasting a week for General Practitioners were established and became very popular, and now continue.

In 1984 the centre was enlarged, giving a much more capacious library and a small seminar room as well as other improvements; the library was named in memory of Mr. A.B. Oliveira. Now the nearby office block is providing an additional seminar room.

The Royal Isle of Wight School of Nursing founded in 1969 had an independent life of about 20 years, - during which time training for S.E.N.s, S.R.N.s and R.M.N.s was carried on. Many of the trainee nurses were Islanders, and there was plenty of local interest, especially perhaps in the annual prize-giving ceremony and award of certificates which was held for several years in the adjacent Isle of Wight College. Numbers, however, were always and inevitably small compared with schools on the mainland and in 1990 it finally ceased to have an independent status and was amalgamated with the Nurse Training School at Portsmouth; nurses may still undergo part of their training at St. Mary's, classes and lectures continue in the Training School now become the School of Health Studies; but it is controlled and managed from Portsmouth; the training of Island midwives has also moved to Portsmouth.

The Patients' services department was developed out of the old Records Department and its headquarters moved to the new hospital when it was opened and Ryde Hospital was closed in 1991. It has a central position in St. Mary's dealing not only with notes but with the arrangements of clinics, the reception of patients; and with lost property, claims for fares and with matters arising from bereavements. It has now a staff of 16. Storage of notes here as elsewhere has presented a problem; the medical staff, aware that *all* our past proclaims our future, would have liked notes to be kept indefinitely; this has not been possible but all notes are kept for a minimum of eight years from the time of the patient's last attendance and some categories are kept longer, indeed some indefinitely. Notes were formerly stored, among other places, in garrets of the House of Industry, in a shed near the entrance to Dodnor Lane which has been replaced by a more modern building for other purposes, and in the tower at Whitecroft. All these have been disused now and notes are stored in the new hospital; this has led to problems and the department has had to borrow space from the adjacent pharmacy which, perhaps unexpectedly, has needed less space than was allowed because of changes in prescribing customs and the amount of work referred to pharmacies outside the hospital.

It has not yet been possible to produce and obtain a diagnostic index, but it is hoped that this will be achieved.

In Ryde the Physiotherapy department established early in the days of the H.M.C. in Partlands Avenue remains the local headquarters with the office of

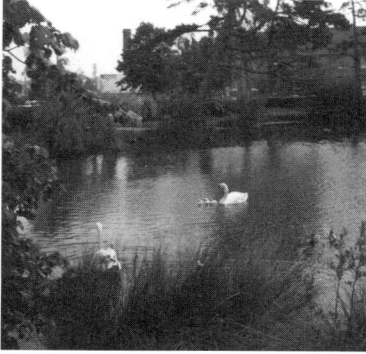

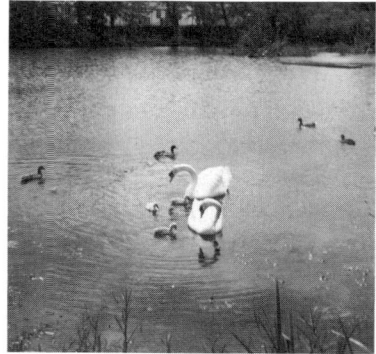

**Plate 17.** 'The Pond' at St. Mary's. The Lower Hospital (Forest House) and the chimney of the boiler-house can be seen through the trees. *Courtesy: Pam Osborne (& others?).*

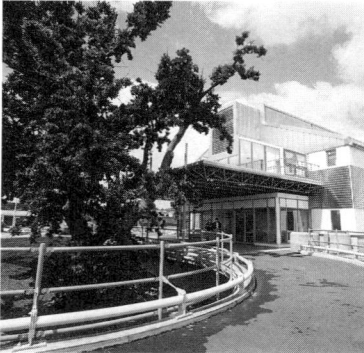

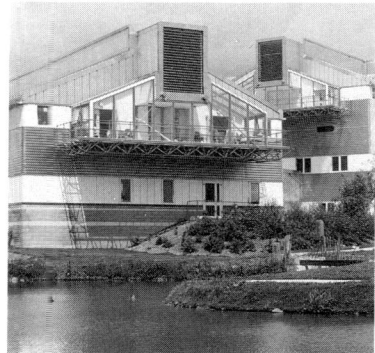

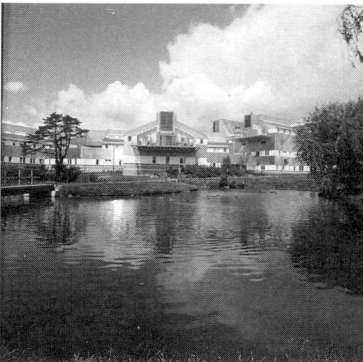

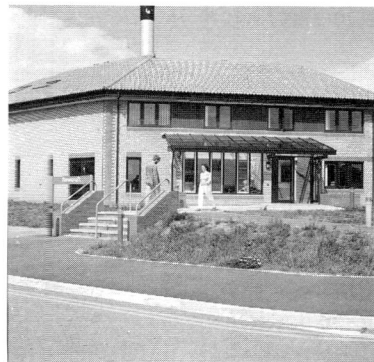

**Plate 18.** Views of the new St. Mary's and Newcroft Hospitals. *Courtesy: J. Bird and Steve Shrimpton of Southampton Teaching Media.*

the Superintendent Physiotherapist; together with the new Out-patient department in Swanmore Road and the nurses' home in Adelaide Place these peripheral components are all that is left now of Ryde Hospital.

In Newport for several years the Physiotherapy Department was established in the old building facing the Forest Road which came to house Forestside School; this was demolished when the relief road was built and the department then had to move to the Upper Hospital where the building of the new kitchens had liberated space hitherto occupied by the kitchens for the Upper Hospital, and the nurses' dining-room. From here up to the time of writing, the physiotherapy services for both the acute and community departments have been organised and managed. I am told that these two elements are shortly to be separated and that one, the acute service, will have to find a new location, but that is not yet history. Trained physiotherapy staff of all grades now number about 20 with about 11 untrained helpers, who receive some in-service training.

The administrative centre for Occupational Therapy is in the large one storey building projecting into the courtyard which used to be the boys' playground; for a long time this building provided training for the mentally handicapped patients in the Lower Hospital. Now the work of about 15 Occupational Therapists is organised here where there is also a wheelchair clinic and where the Speech Therapists and Chiropodists are centred. The Occupational Therapists have a major commitment at Watergate School. Adjacent to this department is the Orthotics workshop occupying a part of the buildings which used to house the mentally disabled men and later was a part of the displaced Barton Ward.

An internal Broadcasting Service was started in 1972, beginning with transmission to one ward, - Ningwood, which has always been closely associated with the Broadcasting Service and remains so now; the service extended in a few years to the whole of St. Mary's. It was, and is, housed on the two floors of the old Chapel of the House of Industry. It is a service run entirely by volunteers. For its equipment it depends upon grants from the hospital and from local and national charities and sponsors; the committee which organises it is elected annually as are the Station Director, the Station Manager and management team. The broadcasters have been trained with Radio Solent and some have gone on to professional appointments with regional and national services. Land lines have been set up to Fairlee and to Frank James Hospitals; these are extremely expensive commodities and to the regret of the service it was never possible to extend it so far as Shanklin Cottage Hospital, but it did reach Whitecroft. The service broadcasts seven days a week between 7.30 a.m. and 10 p.m. with always a request hour between 9 a.m. and 10 a.m.

The idea that patients would feel better and that recovery might be helped by an environment which is attractive, varied and even beautiful rather than dull and drab is not new. In the very early years of Newport Infirmary, the minutes refer to pictures being placed in the wards, and to grants for trees and shrubs in the grounds around them; when the Ministry put a stop to farming and market gardening in hospitals, it still allowed flower gardens and the cultivation of beds and glass houses to provide cut flowers and plants for the wards and other parts of the hospitals; and the new St. Mary's has enclosed gardens onto which some of the wards and corridors look out, and the old pond, still patronised by plenty of ducks and drakes, has been landscaped, and provides a pleasant and desirable contrast from round the corner where, one might say, - Tall grey towers and long steel bars overlook a park of cars. Violet Pilling who was appointed Occupational Therapist at Ryde and Newport briefly before moving to the Royal National Hospital in 1948, was herself a gifted artist and spent at least some of her sessions encouraging and helping patients to divert and amuse themselves by painting and drawing.

The Healing Arts Service is perhaps a further development of these ideas; led by Guy Eades, and established as a charitable activity supported by grants from local and national charities and sponsored by local organisations, it plays an increasing part in promoting recovery and well-being. The department concerns itself with the community as well as the hospital, aiming to stimulate participation in activities such as music, dancing and painting; and is also concerned with the design, decor and furnishing, etc. of the hospital.

Two other institutions related to and arising from the hospital but now independent of it and of the N.H.S. have to be mentioned.

The Hospice movement called for provision for those who could not expect a cure but required treatment and support. Fairlee Hospital had by this time ceased to be needed to any extent for infectious diseases; Dr Graham Thorpe and Mrs. MacGregor, the Matron, especially, urged that it should be put to the use as a Hospice, and after some alterations had been made it was opened in

1982 as a continuing care centre starting with 8 beds. Dr D. Murphy, a consultant physician, who came to the hospital in 1978, supervised it for the first few years with the help especially of Dr Mark Wilks; much additional building and re-modelling has been done and the old Lodge has been incorporated in the Hospice which now provides 12 single rooms with an additional 2 available for sufferers from AIDS, together with reception rooms, day rooms, offices, etc. In 1988 it was re-opened as the Mountbatten Hospice by the Duchess of Kent and became an independent charity; and in 1992 Dr N. Cole was appointed as Medical Director; besides the in-patient beds it provides an out-patient service dealing with about 16 out-patients daily and a Health Information service. It has its own nursing staff with a high nurse/patient ratio and works in conjunction with the three MacMillan nurses. Patients are admitted chiefly for respite care, staying for a few days or a week or two. The Hospice's income is derived in part from a contract with the Health Commission whereby it provides a number of beds for patients referred from the hospital or the community; it also depends upon subscriptions, donations, bequests and its own fund raising activities, and a very successful charity shop in Newport.

The former administrative block at Fairlee Hospital still provides kitchens for the Mountbatten Hospice as well as for Halberry Lodge and some other outlying institutions and part of it is available for a psychology service. Niton Ward has been abandoned being found structurally insecure; and a new building, Halberry Lodge, has been put up on the north side of the central lawn, a psycho-geriatric unit, also independent of the hospital.


The Clinical Allergy Research Unit conceived and founded by Dr David Hide, was for a time accommodated in rooms adjacent to the old restaurant and kitchens; it has now moved to Applegate, near the old entrance to the hospital, which was formerly a house for the Surgical Registrar. It awaits the building of a new department which will be on land to the south of the south hospital, i.e. on the old cricket ground, or what is left of it.

Researches are carried out on food-related and respiratory tract allergy; clinics are held twice weekly and a number of patients with problems of allergy come from the mainland. It is the major pollen and mould recording station for the south of England and broadcasts the tree and grass pollen data throughout the hay fever season and reports to the European Aero-Biology Network.

One new hospital, apart from the new St. Mary's and the new mental hospital - Newcroft, - was built and opened in 1984, the Private Hospital. Lying at the west side of Fairlee Road about half a mile out of Newport, it started with 20 beds, all in single rooms and was later in 1990 enlarged to provide 34 beds. It has an operating theatre, X-ray Department, and Pathology laboratory, although some Pathological work is dealt with in the area laboratory at St. Mary's. Patients from the mainland as well as from the Island are accepted as are children; and self-referred convalescent patients are also admitted. Health screening clinics are provided.

In 1992 the hospital went into receivership, but it did not close, and was sold in 1993 to a consortium of Island men and was renamed the Orchard Hospital; there are now two resident doctors who live in adjacent bungalows belonging to the hospital. Physiotherapy is regularly available and Chiropody and speech therapy can be arranged privately if required.

# XV

## CONCLUSION

In 1952 the Ministry of Health suggested that each H.M.C. should produce yearly a report in narrative form giving account of its activities and development during the year. It would be improperly presumptuous to say that this should have been done; but a would-be historian may perhaps be allowed a passing regret that it was not.

The new hospital was ceremonially opened on September 23rd 1991 by Princess Alexandra; it had been handed over on August 3rd 1990 and it had been occupied in 1990. Newcroft Hospital was occupied in November 1990 and was opened also by Princess Alexandra at a second visit, in December 1991.

With the closure of the Royal County Hospital, many names associated with the hospital have been lost. Cottle, Harington, Milligan, Hathway, Calthorpe, Baring all have vanished. Now it seems that the name of Hassall has followed them into official oblivion. It is perhaps proper to recall the name of A.T.S. Dodd; he was a surgeon who worked about 1840 at the Sussex County Hospital in Chichester; falling ill, he came to Ryde in the hopes of recovery. It was there that he realised the need for a hospital, and with the Rev. Philips, Rector of Newchurch he pioneered its creation, assembling and serving as secretary of the committee which founded it: sadly he died before it was opened.

Since the opening of the new hospitals there has been one other official opening, that of the new Diabetic Centre in what was formerly Seaview Villa very much refurbished and scarcely recognisable. This was carried out by Professor Harry Keen, Chairman of the British Diabetic Association in June 1992.

Of the eleven hospitals which the I.o.W. H.M.C. took over in 1948, plus the one, the Royal National Hospital at Ventnor, which it acquired later, only St. Mary's and the Frank James Hospital remain. Fairlee Hospital - now the Mountbatten Hospice, - is not part of the I.o.W. Trust; there is a new Out-patient department at Ryde adjacent to the hospital and occupying the two houses which had become part of the hospital. The Arthur Webster Institute in Shanklin provides clinics and continues in action. The Royal County Hospital, Whitecroft, the Royal National Hospital, the Ventnor and Undercliff Isolation Hospital, Longford, Ashey, Scio House, and Shanklin Cottage Hospitals, all are gone. Gone too are the military and naval hospitals; Parkhurst Prison Hospital remains and incidentally, in providing an electro-encephalograph service to some degree reciprocates any help which it has received in the past from St. Mary's. The new St. Mary's and Newcroft Hospitals have not however displaced the older St. Mary's; indeed it seems that with the possible exception of the garrets in the oldest buildings of the House of Industry, every corner of St. Mary's is still in use, even the old abandoned pharmacy provides offices; and moreover some new buildings have been added, the Breast Screening unit, and the Renal Dialysis Unit; it is the case however that the Porter's Lodge, the offices connected to it and the former Out-patient, X-ray and records department have been replaced by a car park.

Certain themes seem to run through the story of the hospitals, recurring again and again before and after the National Health Service; no doubt common to all hospitals and all areas; a perpetual shortage of money, or at least an endless demand for more money; staff and managers alike continuously aware of how much more they could do given the means; knowledge and technology always racing ahead of practicalities; long hours spent considering how economies can be achieved or how more money can be extracted from any possible source.

Second only to that perhaps has been the continuing, and never altogether, successful endeavour adequately to accommodate and care for those who in their last few months or years need nursing care, together with the smaller number of unfortunate younger people who must live their days in need of professional help; from the Workhouse to the sick wards, to the Infirmary, and back to the sick wards, - to the medical wards, to the Geriatric wards, to the Part Three Homes and the uneasy partnership with the Social Services, no solution has been entirely sufficient. Surely the concept that the Welfare State would pay for itself through improved health and efficiency was the greatest ever, the supreme, the sublime, miscalculation. Now the attempt to look after the dependants 'in the community', in small and, hopefully, homely homes, is the latest solution; and time will show, statistics apart, whether it is an improvement. One cannot but have the feeling that the problem ever more comes out by the same door as in it went.

This is a murky picture on which to conclude. A very different theme and a far happier one is the continuing relation between the hospital and the community. Hospitals have always, - or almost always - had excellent rapport and relations with the community in which they find themselves, be they large towns (which hardly exist on the Island), small towns, or big villages; the concept of the hospital service has always appealed to the local population which chiefly staffs them. The Christmas shows (and some notable ones have been provided at Ryde, at Whitecroft and at the Royal National Hospital among others), open days, fairs and bazaars have all contributed; the local beneficent organisations, the Red Cross, St. John Ambulance, Toc H, the churches and chapels, Womens' Institutes, Guilds, Buccaneers, Lions, Rotarians and Inner Wheel, Guides and Scouts, and others have all over the years played their part and often a most valuable one, - now supplemented especially by the Friends of the Hospital and more formally by the Community Health Council.

A state service, with its now massive expenditure and numerous personnel is inevitably more formal and remote than before and the more complicated and technically elaborate service requires that complaints and mistakes must be officially recognised, discussed and reported and tribute is due to Mr. Lewis and his assistants for their work in dealing with such matters; but I believe that despite all the formality and the extensive super-structure needed for managing the hospital, those going into St. Mary's or Frank James or elsewhere for treatment generally still feel that they are in the hands of friends and that their hospital is ready and glad to receive and help them. If this be true and fair comment, then all may be well. Antonia Fraser in *Cromwell, Our Chief of Men* records that Catherine Viscountess Ranelagh, sister of Robert Boyle, the great physicist, and friend of Milton, wrote 'Me-thinks every contrivance, tending to the care of the sick, or the welfare of mankind under any part of that curse he groans under, may be an exercise of love ...'. If this be the belief which inspires all those who work in any and every part of the service, it must surely succeed. But is it?

# Abbreviations used in the Text or the Index

| | | | |
|---|---|---|---|
| A & E | Accident & Emergency | L.G.B. | Local Government Board |
| A.H.A. | Area Health Authority | MoH | Medical Officer of Health |
| C.M.O. | County Medical Officer | M.O.H. | Ministry of Health |
| C.S.S.D. | Central Sterile Supply | N.H.S. | National Health Service |
| | Department | O.T. | Occupational Therapy |
| D.H.A. | District Health Authority | P.A.C. | Public Assistance Committee |
| E.C.T. | Electro-convulsion Therapy | P.L.B. | Poor Law Board |
| E.N.T. | Ear, Nose & Throat | RIoWCH | Royal Isle of Wight County |
| E.S.M.I. | Elderly Severely Mentally Ill | | Hospital |
| H of I | House of Industry | R.M.N. | Registered Mental Nurse |
| H.M.C. | Hospital Management | R.N.H. | Royal National Hospital |
| | Committee | S.M. | Saint Mary's (Hospital) |

# INDEX

County, Medical Officer 131
    see also Dr Walker: Dr Fairley: Dr
    Wallace: Dr Machell: Dr Henderson
    Press (Newspaper) 9, 77
Cowper, Dr 119
Cross, Miss 53
Crosskey, Dr 159, 174
Curtis (Builder) 29
Cutler, T.W., F.R.I.B.A. 27

Dabbs, Dr 119, 120
Dabell, Mr 76, 129
Daish, W.G. 45
Darmady, Dr 46, 153
Dash, George 21, 24, 41, 42
Davey, Dr 27, 42
Davies-Jones, Dr 103, 153
Davis, Major, R.A.M.C. 135
Dentist & Dental Surgeons 42, 45, 75,
    134, 159, 180, 185
Diabetic Centre 82, 184, 197
Directors of House of Industry 62, 64
Dispensaries 14, 29, 163, 166
    see also Pharmacy
District Health Authority 177 et seq.
Dobie, Mrs. 29
Dobson, Dr S. 154
Dockray, Dr J. 39, 46, 150, 153, 158
Doctors on the IoW 13
Dodd, Dr A.T.S. 18, 197
Drainage 24, 27, 69, 82

Eade, F.L.W. 150, 176
Eades, Guy 194
East Cowes Hospital
    see Frank James Hospital
Easton, Dr 111, 113, 114
Ebbisham, Lord 107
    Ward 109
Edwards, W. 155, 183
Eldridge, James 17
Eliot, T.S. (Ward) 173, 175
Elizabeth (Ward) 31
Emergency Medical Service 39, 53, 134

E.N.T. Dept. 36, 153
Erskine, Dr 101, 102
Eversley, Lord 107
    Ward 109

Fairlee Hospital 123, 129 et seq. 158, 194,
    197
Fairley, Dr 39, 91, 92, 131, 133, 164
Farms & Gardens 99, 105, 107, 150, 151
Finances (Ryde) 49 et seq.
Finch, Dr 68
Firman-Edwards, Dr 45, 46, 153, 156, 157
Fleming, Baldwyn 74, 76, 79
Forest House 60, 76, 87
    see also H of I & St. Mary's Hospital
Forest-Side School 75, 156
Frank James Hospital 115 et seq, 133, 155,
    174, 175
Frank Linsly James 115
Friend, Miss 37

Gardiner, Col. 53
Garlick & Horton (Builders) 97
Gaynor, Mr. (Surgeon) 121, 152
George V Memorial, Home
    see Nurses' Home
    Wing
    see Frank James Hospital
Geriatric, Day Hospital 171
    Department 158, 168, 186
Glynn, P. (Chairman) 85
Golden Hill Fort & Hospital 141
Gordon, Mr. (Secretary) 39
Governors, RIoWCH 17, 32 et seq.
    House of Industry 61, 68
    see also Master
Gregor, S. (Architect) 103
Griffin, W. (Dental Surgeon) 45
Grimaldi, Philip 145, 153, 159
Groves, Dr 29

Hall, Stanley (Architect) 30
Hambrough, J. 19
Hamilton Fund 108